Holistic Nursing

Holism and Holistic Health Care for Nurses

By

Nirjharini Tripathy

Holistic Nursing

Copyright © 2019

ISBN: 9781698628639

Warning and Disclaimer

Publisher contact

Skinny Bottle Publishing

books@skinnybottle.com

Part One

All about Holistic Nursing

Introduction

Every human being is more than merely a sum of his or her parts. Who better to know the very same, other than the modern nurse?

In fact, that's the very reason there is a pivotal need for holistic nursing. Truth be told, holistic nursing is more than merely the apparently integrated approach that most modern nurses take towards their patients. More than anything, it's a way of life. The philosophy and way of thinking that comprise the very tenets of holistic nursing, is intrinsically incorporated into the lives of the nurses. It becomes a part of their professional life and more importantly, their identity.

In the mid-19th century, Florence Nightingale revolutionized the role of the modern nurse by incorporating the very holistic approach that is seen in the work of so many modern nurses in today's day and age. No longer was nursing merely working towards healing the body, but towards enriching the human spirit as well. It's the human spirit, really, that needs to be fortified if one needs to find some tangible improvement in the condition of the body, and this is exactly what Florence Nightingale set out to establish, thus laying the foundation for what is generally accepted as the modern practice of holistic healing today.

In fact, the very premise of holistic healing is based on treating the mind, body, and soul as a whole. Yes, nursing in the middle ages was becoming somewhat mechanized, with the increased use of machines and medicines. What had happened prior to the Florence Nightingale era was the fact that nursing had lost that most pivotal sense of human contact that is so essential in bringing about some tangible change in recovery in so many patients who have lost the will to survive. There was an increasing need to bring back that sense of humanity into the practice, and that is what led to the modern holistic approach we find in nursing today.

The main tenet in holistic nursing is the fact that every human being is a different person, and as such needs to be treated differently from others. That is the way they can heal in a way like no other. For instance, there might be people who have an inherent faith in God, and yet others who find music to be deeply relaxing. Have you ever wondered if music might play a pivotal role in relaxing a person succinctly enough before his or her surgery? Well, it can and that is exactly what a nurse trained well in the holistic approach, might recommend. It doesn't end there, either. After the surgery, they might even ask the patient if they would like aromatherapy or perhaps even a massage, in order to help them feel better.

In this book, you will literally get a hands-on, holistic approach to finding out what exactly holistic nursing is all about. Let's get started then, shall we, and delve into the wonderful world of holistic nursing without further ado.

Chapter 1

What is Holistic Nursing?

Holistic nursing in its primordial essence is a specialty in nursing that is concerned with the integration of a person's mind, body, and spirit with their environment. It focuses on the mind, body, and spirit working together as a whole, and how spiritual awareness in nursing can help to heal illness. Therefore, the primary focus of holistic nursing is to heal the entire patient.

In fact, the principles of holistic nursing have come from no other than the great Florence Nightingale herself – the principles of holism: *unity, wellness and the interrelationship of human beings and their environment.*

In the year 2006, the American Nursing Association (ANA) officially recognized holistic nursing as a specialty of nursing practice. The very origins of a nursing association with a view to promoting holistic healing in patients started with the foundation of the American Holistic Nurses Association (AHNA) way back in 1980. This organization was founded with the view to promote the education of nurses and others in the philosophy, practice, and research of holistic care and healing.

So, in her very essence, a holistic nurse is nothing short of being a nurse who takes the mind-body-spirit-emotion-environment approach and applies it in the practice of traditional modern nursing. She recognizes and integrates the principles and modalities of holistic healing into daily life and clinical practice. In fact, holistic nursing gives a spiritual boost to nurses themselves and helps them incorporate spirituality into their very own lives. This, in turn, leads them to have greater empathy towards the souls they treat (for the patients they are treating are now looked at as more than ephemeral bodies with minds). Now, they are treating the trinity of body, mind, and soul and that is what makes their work all the more magnanimous.

Florence Nightingale might have very well been the pioneer of what we know today as the modern holistic healing approach that is used by so many nurses worldwide, but it has indeed come a long way since then. What is not going to change, however, is the fact that people will continue to fall sick. The really great thing holistic nursing has done is ensure that every patient is not seen merely as a patient or a diagnosis. They are not merely to be treated with medicines and machines so that the nurse can move on to the next patient in a near robotic fashion. The whole process of holistic nursing as detailed as taking into consideration the social and cultural differences and preferences of the individual patient. The emphasis here is on the word individual, as every person is just that: *an individual that is worthy of individual care.* The idea is for the nurse to take her time with the patient, rather than merely rushing on in an attempt to get to the next one.

No wonder then, that holistic nurses are seen by their patients as the ones that 'truly care'. And why shouldn't they? After all, they truly do.

The Philosophy behind Holistic Healing

The Holistic Healing philosophy is based on the belief that every person, on the whole, is made up of interdependent parts and if one part is not working properly, then all the other parts will be affected. So, if people have physical, emotional or even spiritual imbalances in their lives, it can have an adverse impact on their overall health.

The idea here is that health is really an overall state of being, with all these components playing an important part. Sometimes these components are well aligned with one another, and sometimes, well, they are simply misaligned. The fact of the matter is that the body, mind, and soul work in conjunction with each other to facilitate the whole system that forms the person. When this system is in flow, energy flows naturally through the body, without any blockages or restrictions. On the other hand, when it is out of the flow, the energy accumulates and as a result, there is a stagnation of energy.

So, the reason that holistic healing works is that when we approach life from all its aspects – *the physical, emotional and spiritual*, what we are really doing, in essence, is leaving no area uncovered – no area of the system we are fine-tuning in order to get the best possible results. Therefore, the healing process is far greater where it comes to holistic healing because change is happening on all those three levels – physical, emotional and spiritual. Therefore, the positive changes that occur in the process are more likely to last long-term and improve the overall quality of life of the patient.

The philosophy behind holistic healing is to avoid the 'Band-Aid fix' approach of conventional nursing and look beyond the person's physical state and see their holistic being or functioning. It is the latter that needs to be treated, and therefore one might be able to solve some problems that were hitherto irresolvable when treated with conventional medicine. It is now widely recognized that the root cause of a physical illness might actually be non-physical, thanks to the emergence of holistic healing.

Therefore, what holistic healing proposes to do is restore that vital sense of balance that is missing from a person when he or she is not keeping the best of health. It's true that when an organ is out of balance, we feel something is wrong and we want things to be like they were before. We want to return to that natural state of harmony, where everything works as intended. This process of rebalancing, really, is nothing short of being synonymous with the process of healing. In fact, the very definition of healing is *'Bringing any imbalance into alignment with its natural state of functioning'*.

16

So, the basic principle behind holistic healing is wholeness. When we can achieve that sense of wholeness by respecting all the components of our system – the physical, emotional and spiritual, we can be complete. We can be whole.

What makes us Whole?

Before we delve into the intricacies of Holistic Nursing, it's only prudent to take a closer look at what exactly makes us human beings *whole* – that very whole that we constantly aspire to preserve over time, thus enabling us to live happy, fulfilling lives.

There are various aspects that must be taken into consideration when we are considering wholeness. Some of them are as follows:

Having the utmost respect for our bodies

Healing our relationship

Caring for the environment

When we talk about health in general, we are really talking about three types of health. They are the physical, mental and spiritual. The problem here is that we often treat each one of them separately, as though they might not be related. For instance, we might see a psychologist for our mental health and a healer, for our spiritual needs.

Is it really possible, though, to separate that mental health from our spiritual health? Or, for that matter, our physical health from our mental health? The truth is a resoundingNo; they are all really interconnected.

A lot of times, having a holistic approach to life has been confused with being spiritual. Although spirituality might indeed be an important component of holistic well being, it is important to realize that it is only one of the three components. Holistic well being also about doing things like eating clean so that our body can be in the prime of health. It also means that we have to play a great deal of attention to our emotional framework, as we all know how terrible we can feel when those emotions go out of whack.

Being whole furthermore means that we must always strive to grow in our lives. We must seek a higher purpose, and always strive to be better than we already are. This does not mean only in the spiritual sense; it means that we should always aspire towards learning things that can add to our lives.

When we have a deep sense of gratitude in our lives, that goes a long way towards making us whole. Instead of constantly fretting over the things we don't have, we come to realize that there are so many things in our lives that we need to be grateful for. That helps us love life to the fullest and makes us happy and whole.

On the way to being whole, you will find that there are many people that you will meet along the way, who will help you. They will naturally come into your life, but you can make an attempt to find them as well.

You will also find that the ingredients of patience, love, and kindness will help greatly in making you whole. They will help you become more awake as a person, and help take your life to the heights you were destined to grace. You will have better relations with the people around you and an enriching life you can enjoy to the fullest.

The Basics – What is Health?

All this while we have been talking about the holistic approach to health. However, do we even realize what the word health even means? It's integral to get a pivotal sense of the same before we begin our holistic journey ahead. Let's take a look, then, at what health really means in the fullest sense.

The truth is, health is more than ephemerally a good or bad feeling, or an aesthetic look. It is really the all-encompassing state of who we people are as individuals.

As discussed earlier, health can be divided into three components: physical, mental and spiritual. However, do we even know what each of these really encompasses? Let's take a look.

Physical Health

Physical health is the state your bodily systems and structures are in at any given point in time. When your physical health has gone awry you will be prone to experience symptoms internally as well as externally. These symptoms can include pain and rashes; anything, really, that manifests itself physically on or within your body.

19

Mental Health

This can also be referred to as *emotional health*. It refers to the condition of your mind and the ability to balance emotions. It includes how you respond to stress. A lot of times people are aware of their poor mental health, but might not be willing to do anything to correct it. Mental health issues, however, are as important as those of the physical kind and certainly nothing to be ashamed of.

Spiritual Health

This component of health is often misconstrued as being confused with being religious. While spiritual people might also be religious, spirituality and religion are not the same. Spiritual health has really more to do with your morals and values, and how they influence the direction your life takes. It involves you being able to discern between what is right and what is wrong and to question the very fabric of your existence.

When we look at health as being comprised of these three components, another important thing is clear. That health *is not merely the absence of disease*. You might have a devastating physical ailment like cancer but it is how you respond to it that determines your overall health. You could remain defeated and lose all sense of hope, or you could rise like a phoenix from the ashes on account of your inherently strong spiritual self and still manage to find happiness in the face of that impending chaos.

The good news when you look at health from all angles, thus, is the fact that you might not always be able to attain perfect health, but you can surely be healthy partially. Of course, the goal always remains to strive towards wellness on the whole. However, you can rest assured your health is not completely in the doldrums and you are stronger than you might have otherwise thought. *You might not be whole on the whole, but you can certainly be whole in part!*

Chapter 2

The Key Principles to Holistic Healing

It's time to take a step forward and delve deeper into our pursuit of finding out exactly all that holistic healing entails. Let's take a look, then, at the key principles to holistic healing so that we can get a keener understanding of the same.

Maintaining good health is more than merely taking care of your physical body

Let's consider the hypothetical situation where you have a headache that just doesn't seem to go away. What do you do? You visit the doctor, only to come back with an over the counter prescription for headache medicine. Instead of merely treating the problem, did you consider doing something to get to the root of the problem, like getting better sleep? You might even try to assess the day and look for stress triggers that might be the very cause of that headache. When you have a holistic approach, you treat yourself on the whole and not merely the problem that you are experiencing.

Holistic health involves treating the emotional component

It's true; a lot of physical ailments have their roots in emotional causes. You will find that when you are able to do things like surround a patient with his family and near and dear ones, you will be doing a really great job where it comes to aiding in the healing process and helping the patient get back to their normal state.

Alternative Medicine can be used, but not always exclusively

What is alternative medicine anyways? Well, any sort of medicine that is considered unorthodox by the medical community. Some of the more famous examples of this kind of medicine include *herbalism, homeopathy, and acupuncture.* Of course, a holistic practitioner might even use conventional medicine, but the important thing to bear in mind here is that he or she is treating *the cause of the problem and not merely the symptoms.*

Holistic healing involves how we deal with our environment

23

You will find that we all have the innate ability to heal ourselves. For instance, if you have some stress about something coming up, it might manifest into that headache we talked about earlier. Now, you might go on and make things worse by increasing your caffeine intake, or you could instead make smart food and exercise choices and in turn get rid of that headache, after all.

The Healing Power of Love

Love is all-important and you will find that holistic health care practitioners strive to meet the patient's needs without any conditions, using *grace, kindness, and awareness* that all stem from knowing that the greatest healer, in the end, is love.

Unity of Body, Mind, and Spirit

Last but certainly not the least, holistic health care practitioners view people on the whole as being integrations of body, mind, and spirit and the focus, as such, is treating a person on the whole and not merely the parts he or she is composed of.

Chapter 3

Holistic Healing – How It Works

Let's take a look at how the process of holistic healing actually works, by examining what it is that actually makes us healthy in the very first place.

What makes us healthy – the different levels of being

So, what is the elixir to life? What is it that can be said to be responsible for the healthy state of an individual? Let's take a more intimate look at the different levels of being, so we can understand exactly what it is that makes us healthy.

Physical Wellness

25

Of course, the very first thing that comes to our minds when we think about the term wellness is physical health. It really goes without saying that the overall state of our bodies is responsible for our good health and well being. So, what exactly are the components of physical wellbeing? Roughly speaking, they are as follows.

What makes us physically healthy

The implementation of regular physical activity. Exercise those blues away.

The maintenance of a healthy diet. Eating right

The rejuvenation of our bodies through rest and sleep. They told you to get eight hours of sleep, right? They weren't kidding.

Emotional Wellness

The number one killer out there, really, is stress. Stress is the cause of the entire emotional imbalance in our lives, and if left untreated it can get to a point where it can even become debilitating. According to the study *Stress in America* undertaken by the American Psychological Association in 2015, more than 40 percent of adults are lying awake at night on account of stress. In fact, stress is responsible for various other crippling conditions like anxiety and heart disease. So, how exactly do we counteract the negative effects of this stress in our lives?

What makes us emotionally healthy

Getting into a fixed routine. Our adrenal glands thrive on predictability. If you go to bed at the same time every night and wake up at the same time every morning, you will find that you are able to succinctly keep those stress demons at bay.

Seeking support from a mental health care professional. Sometimes, when you are not able to cope on your own, this is the best thing to do. There's nothing to be ashamed of, really.

Spiritual Wellness

The spiritual life is the life that we live inside ourselves, apart from the lives that we live outside ourselves. You will find that if you are spiritually rich, it is really worth more than all the material treasures in the world. So, how exactly do we achieve this profound spiritual bliss?

One of the best possible things to make us spiritually healthy would be to meditate. Meditation can be one of the most effective ways to get in touch with your spiritual side. All you have to do, really, is to give yourself that me time in the day, where you will find yourself capable of fostering feelings of deep peace and relaxation, by simply zoning out and focusing on what is the naked, real you. You don't have to meditate for long; all it really takes is five minutes daily, and you will be amazed at the change.

How Holistic Recuperation works – How do we get into alignment?

So, you must be curious by now, to see how the process of holistic recuperation really works, right? What is that magical process through which we get into alignment with the selves we are now mere fragments of? Let's take a look at the same, so we understand exactly how we can live the lives we were intended to.

The fact of the matter is, there are so many different things happening all the time – things we are not really aware of on a conscious level. Even though we might not be conscious of the same, these life situations cause us to respond physically, emotionally and spiritually, all at the same time.

We have already seen that the process of holistic healing involves the three components – the physical, mental and spiritual.

What happens over time, then, is this: each and every small thing that the body, mind or soul resists accumulates, and we tend to get further and further out of alignment with our true selves. Then, even if we are out of alignment on only one of the three levels, over time it might tantamount to us feeling discomforted, or plain and simply unhealthy.

It is this very feeling of being in a state of discord, that seeks us to bridge the gap and somehow make an attempt to get ourselves aligned again, thus setting the stage for that all-important process of holistic recuperation. So, how does holistic recuperation really work?

There are in essence two primordial goals of holistic healing

To balance each level

To balance all levels with each other

All we have to do, really, is to focus on the first step as when this is achieved (i.e. when all the levels are balanced), the three levels will automatically align with each other. That is when you shall find, that the state of wholeness is achieved.

So, what is the approach that is used to ensure that the process of holistic recuperation takes place?

The answer lies in the word, *purification*. It is when purification on all levels of being is achieved, that energy flows freely through all systems without any blockages or restrictions. In time we become more sensitive to these imbalances and are able to correct them at will.

The goal here, then, would be to have a balanced lifestyle that would help to get all those levels into a state of balance. In fact, a lot of us tend to live with at least one level off balance. Some are even living their lives with all levels out of balance, while yet others are in a state of perfect alignment. By now you know what to do when you are out of balance, right? That's right – all you have to do is get into that natural state of balance again. Then you will find what you have been missing out on all this while. And, of course, it will be well worth it.

Chapter 4

Holism and Holistic Nursing

Now that we have understood the basic principles of holistic healing, it's time to take a nosedive into the area that we will be dissecting in great detail over the course of this book – how the process of holism applies to holistic nursing, that is. Let's take a look at some of the key tenets of holism where it comes to the most dignified profession of holistic nursing.

The Practitioner – Patient Relationship

The fact of the matter is, nursing is a tough profession. It can be physically, mentally and spiritually draining at times. This is the very reason that at times nurses feel rushed and cannot spend quality time with their patients. On the other hand, there are those moments of magic that they spend with their patients, that really serves to remind them what nursing is all about.

That is where holistic nursing steps in. It's not really about the amount of time that one spends with a patient, but rather the quality of time spent with them. When a nurse promotes a patient's well being, you will find that they can dramatically alter their rate of improvement. The relationship between them and the patient changes, and you will find that it leads to better patient outcomes which in turn increases the levels of happiness and sense of purpose in the nurses themselves.

So, what then are the key tenets of a practitioner-patient relationship? Briefly put, they are the following.

The Key Tenets of the Practitioner – Patient relationship

Learning the patient's name and using it

Maintaining that sense of eye contact with the patient at all times

Sincerely asking the patient how they are feeling

Using the beauty of the smile and laughing when appropriate

Using the therapeutic power of touch

Empowering the patient to see themselves as being worthy of dignity

Preserving that very dignity of the patients

Educating the patients on the value of self-care

Asking the patients how one can relive their pain and anxiety

Using highly effective, non-pharmacological methods of pain control like imagery and relaxation techniques

Assisting the patients with alternative treatments like massage, aromatherapy, and music, if needed

Asking the patients if they have any spiritual or religious beliefs and being sensitive and caring about them if they do.

In the end, it's really not all about how many holistic actions the nurse can perform for patients. It's really all about the quality of time that they spent with them, having the intention to care for each patient as a whole and really caring to be with that patient. There is absolutely no healthcare setting out there where holistic nursing cannot be provided.

The underlying idea here is that every person is an individual, and as such the practitioner-patient relationship must also be an individual one, to ensure that only the best possible care is provided for the patient. It's not about not being task-oriented or goal-oriented, it's simply to ensure that you strike the right balance, and bring that much-needed sense of balance into the patient's life.

Practitioner – Community Relationship

It must be noted that nurses can become excellent advocates for the communities in which we live, thanks to patient advocacy and excellent service delivery. They are in fact the front-line witnesses to countless patient experiences, and thereby have great scope to improve public well-being through legislative activism. There are different strategies by which nurse practitioners can become excellent advocates for their patients. Let's have a look at some of them.

Participation in community assessments.

By participating in community assessments, nurse practitioners can help ensure that officials gather the relevant information that can help bring about positive change. Some of these bits of information are the following.

Population Age distributions

Community health conditions

Economic obstacles

Employment statistics

Ethnic group populations

Health care service performance levels

Housing conditions

It must be noted that these bits of information are collected cyclically by government officials, with a view to maintaining continual community well-being.

Civic Interest Group formation

Nurse practitioners play a pivotal role in community mentorship and networking. You will find that they can facilitate ongoing community partnerships to manage current health issues. These activities allow the nurse practitioners to establish community initiatives that continually foster the caregiver talent within a particular locale.

Advocacy for cost-effective treatments and medications

There are many stakeholders in the health care field, who can affect change through legislation. The legislators must review the evidence carefully and make the decisions that are in the best interests of the public. Therefore, it is critical that nurse practitioners voice the needs of the patrons of the community, through the legislative process.

Maintaining Rapport with Academic Influencers

Nurse practitioners can succinctly establish the rapport that allows them to be effective advocates of student health, by continually educating administrators, students and parents about community wellness issues. This sustained relationship allows them to establish a rapport with the people that monitor and advocate for concerns like ensuring sufficient nurse staffing levels in schools. By maintaining an ongoing sense of rapport with the people who are involved in academic decision making, they can advocate for the patient's needs as and when it is required.

Involvement with Local Organizations

There is a great deal of competition that exists between local organizations where it comes to rallying for general funding. Here you will find that the nursing professionals out there can actually fight for the best programs that will serve the best interests of the people because they are continually abreast of all the latest happenings in the field. They can effectively identify key public health resources, services, and issues.

Public Education

You will find that nurse practitioners can maintain community relations by providing ongoing wellness education. This helps in turn to build their reputation as health care experts. It also helps to promote a dialogue that involves local residents and community health concerns. This brings together practitioners and patients and ensures heightened community involvement in its health care future. This helps make nurse practitioners in the workplace highly informed community health advocates.

Chapter 5

Self Care with Holistic Nursing

It is absolutely imperative to understand that self-care is integral where it comes to one's personal health, the sustenance to continue to care for others and in the area of professional growth. There is, therefore, an increasing need to practice self-care so as to combat stress and promote health in practice.

Of course, nurses are far more effective when they themselves are able to maintain solid physical, mental and spiritual health. The really unfortunate thing is, because these nurses are so selflessly committed to looking after the needs of others, they can often let their very own needs go neglected. Let's take a look, then, at how one can perform the most effective self-care in the holistic nursing arena.

Areas for Self-Care for Nurses

Before we can take a look at how self-care can be effectively incorporated into the holistic nursing experience, let's take a look at the different areas that need to be touched upon, where it comes to achieving those exalted levels of self-care.

Hygiene (this includes general and personal)

Nutrition (the type and quality of food eaten)

Lifestyle (sporting activities and leisure)

Environmental factors (living conditions and social habits)

Socioeconomic factors (income levels and cultural beliefs)

Self-medication

The whole idea of self-care is to embody those very values that one wishes to see in one's patients. For instance, if a nurse is healthy and enjoys life, they will be all the more empowered to bring about the same qualities in their patients.

Let's take a look at some really great self-care tips for nurses

Self-care tips for nurses with a view to promoting effective holistic healthcare

Physical

Make sure that healthy food is incorporated into the daily diet. To make sure that exercise is incorporated into one's daily routine. It does not have to be all that elaborate like going to a gym; all one really needs is to use that lunch break to go for a walk. One needs to get more active and instead of sitting at the nurses' station all the while, one could walk the hallways looking out for their patients.

Intellectual

The brain must also be treated like a muscle that needs to be flexed regularly in order to keep it sharp. So, doing things like keeping up on nursing journals and magazines and making suggestions for change, can all help to benefit the intellectual stimulation process.

Emotional

One must keep their own emotions in check at all times. Everyone has bad days. It's perfectly all right and what matters is to keep your chin up and keep going no matter what.

Spiritual

One can add mindfulness activities like yoga and mindfulness meditation, to their working week in order to calm the mind and get more in touch with their spiritual selves. One might even wish to engage in a faith or perhaps even spiritual community. That will surely go a long way in empowering them spiritually.

Chapter 6

Holistic Communication – Creating a therapeutic environment

The surroundings that we are in at any given point in time have such a great influence on our selves as a whole. Why not, then, create the perfect environment for healing itself? Let's take a look at what it takes to create that very healing surrounding.

Growing a Healing Surrounding

Cultivating a therapeutic environment depends on several factors. Here are some of the more important ones.

Making the hospital as quiet as possible

Of course, it goes without saying that a hospital is the place where people go to heal. How is one supposed to heal in peace when there is sound all the time, even in the wee hours of the night? There must be a great degree of care that is undertaken to ensure that the hospital is as quiet as possible, in order to help the patients heal in the best manner possible.

Having single-bed rooms

You wouldn't share your hotel room with a stranger; why then would you share your hospital room with one? It's really a matter of the issue of personal hygiene, where it comes to the same. The last thing you want is to get an infection from your neighbor. In fact, the trend over the last few years has seen fewer people being grouped alongside each other in hospital rooms. Let's hope the day is not far off when there will be a single bedroom available for every patient.

Staffing ratios

Oftentimes the very reason we find that adequate nursing care is not given to patients is on account of the fact that there are simply not enough nurses to handle the number of patients in the hospital. One must certainly think of expanding their budget and providing more staff for their patients, especially when it will have a tangible benefit of showing great results and thereby upping the reputation of the institution in the process. In the end, you want *happy patients*, don't you?

Hospital design

The last thing you want is a place that makes you feel queasy, no matter where you are. If you're in a nice hotel, you will know it instantly. The same applies to hospitals.

You want to feel you are in a nice setting; one that is indeed therapeutic enough to make you heal well. Therefore, a lot of thought must go into designing hospitals, be it external design or internal design. There must be as much open space incorporated as possible, and a great level of attention must be paid to minute details like the hospital flooring.

Taking patients outside the room

You will find that those patients that are merely cooped up in their hospital beds for too long have lower levels of motivation than those who are regularly ferreted out for a stroll or two. The latter group recover better and faster, and also have a lower risk for deep vein thrombosis (which is a clot in the leg).

The Holistic Caring Process

The Holistic Caring process, therefore, in lieu of a therapeutic environment, would be to create the perfect environment for the patient in which he or she will be able to fully recover to the very best of their abilities. There are many factors that aid the implementation of a truly great holistic caring system. Let's have a look at the same.

Self-care

Educating patients and helping them become independent enough to perform their own self-care on a daily basis, in order to get them independent and therein finally break the cords of dependency so that they can rely on the best people who can ultimately provide care for them – their very own selves.

Speech

Holistic communication through speech. When words are spoken to the patient by the nursing professional, they must be spoken in a slow manner, ensuring that the words are enunciated properly. The choice of words spoken, too, must be those that are easy to understand and not all that technical. Care must be taken to only present the most relevant information, so as to avoid any sense of confusion.

Non-verbal

Non-verbal messages or signals should be used in order to get the message across without the usage of words. These can be divided into several categories, like *facial expressions, gestures and body language*. Even something like the physical appearance of the nurse can have a great impact on the state of the patient. The intonation of the voice should be soft so that it will be pleasing to the ears. A simple facial expression like a heartfelt smile can go a long way in garnering that sense of trust and confidence in a patient.

Written communication

This is also an important form of holistic communication that needs to be taken seriously. You will find that when things are to be written, they need to be done in a manner that is complete and concise. There should, therefore, be no kind of ambiguity when one is preparing things like records, reports, and policies. If there is any kind of ambiguity, the problem that ensues can result in a great deal of misunderstanding.

Holistic communication

It is essential for providing the right holistic caring environment, and there is one way in which you will find out whether communication has indeed been effective or not. When the receiver of the communication reacts, then he or she is the communicator. When that communication is akin to the sort of communication the communicator expected from the receiver, then it is a given that the communication has hit the nail on the head.

Active listening

This also plays a great role in holistic communication. You will find the key to effective communication lies not only in getting one's message across to the receiver but also actively playing a part in listening to what the receiver has to say. This will only serve to provide the best therapeutic environment for the patient, who knows the caregiver actually has a strong sense of empathy for them.

There are some basic tenets of the holistic caring process that one has to bear in mind. These are the following.

The Assessment Process

In this stage, you will find that the nurses assess each person holistically using the appropriate conventional and holistic methods, while at the same time honoring the uniqueness of the person. In this stage, you will find that the process of holistic assessment includes the appropriate traditional and holistic methods in order to systematically gather information. The holistic nurse here strives to value all types of knowledge while gathering data from a person and goes on to gather this information and validate it with intuitive knowledge, where deemed appropriate.

Patterns/Challenges/Needs

You will find that holistic nurses prioritize and identify each person's actual and potential patterns/challenges/needs and the life patterns that are related to health, wellness, disease or illness, that might or might not facilitate wellbeing. It is here that the nurses will partner with the person in a mutual decision process in order to create a health care plan for each pattern/challenge/need that there is, or the opportunity to enhance health and well being. It also helps a person to identify the areas for education to make decisions about life choices in a conscious and informed manner that empowers the person to maintain his or her uniqueness and independence. It also helps them to offer self-association tools, word associations, and storytelling as appropriate. You will come to see that the holistic nurses use skills of cultural competence and communicate the acceptance of the person's values, beliefs, culture, and even socioeconomic background. They also serve to help the person to recognize at-risk patterns/challenges/needs for potential or existing health situations (like family health history and age-related health risk factors), and assist in recognizing opportunities in order to enhance well being. They encourage the person in problem-solving dialogue in relation to changes secondary to illness and treatment.

Implementation

In this stage, you will find that holistic nurses prioritize each person's plan of holistic care, and the holistic caring interventions are planted in accordance with the same. Here, the holistic nurses help implement the mutually created plan of care within the context of assisting the person within the higher context of health and well being. They also go on to support and promote the person's capacity for the highest level of participation and problem-solving where it comes to the health care plan and also collaborate with the other team members where deemed appropriate. They thus use their holistic nursing skills in implementing care, including cultural competency and all ways of knowing. They advocate that the person's plan and unique healing process be honored, and provide the care that is clear about and respectful of, the economic parameters of practice, striving to balance justice with compassion.

Evaluation

In this stage, you will find that the holistic nurses will evaluate each person's response to holistic care regularly and systematically, and recognize and honor the continuous holistic nature of the healing process. The following are the steps where it comes to a thorough holistic evaluation. Firstly, they collaborate with the person as well as with the other health care team members when appropriate, in the process of evaluating the holistic outcomes. Next, they will explore with the person his or her explanation of the cause of any significant sort of deviation that might be there between the responses and the expected outcomes. They will also mutually create with the person and the other team members, a revised plan if so needed.

Part 2

Holistic Nursing and the Transpersonal Self

Introduction

It is important to remember that the act of synchronizing the mind and the body is not something that has been randomly called into existence. It is, in fact, a basic principle of the human spirit: the integration of the mind, body, and spirit, that is.

You will find that throughout the course of history, there has been a quest and a universal need to understand why there is human life in the very first instance, as well as what happens after we die.

Nurses have to evolve to their highest potential and go beyond their limited selves, to what is known as their transpersonal selves. When they can do that, they can truly understand the dimensions of healing themselves as well as others. You will find that the very body of this knowledge is perennial philosophy. The roots of this philosophy are found in all traditional lore, right from the most primitive, to the most highly developed cultures in the world.

A person's wholeness and healing are determined by the awareness on all the levels. You will find here that the Absolute Self is that which transcends everything and also includes everything. Now, as nurses reflect on the inner dimension of the Self and ways of Being, this conscious journey towards wholeness evolves towards the pursuit of self-transcendence. You will find that early on in the process of our ego development, self-consciousness arises as a prerequisite for healthy human development. You will find, however, that as the self continues to develop and mature, the different *self-concepts, identities and personal experiences* lead towards the pivotal conscious journey of inner understanding.

The psyche is observed to have many layers and as one moves inwards, seeking inner knowledge and personal understanding, one goes on to experience the *Absolute* that is composed of higher-ordered wholes as well as integrations. It must be noted here that the basic structures of the psyche are not replaced, but rather become a part of the larger unity. You will find here that the ultimate part of the journey is enlightening, or the awakening to the knowledge that the one is really a part of the whole.

Within the discipline of nursing, there is a widespread acceptance of the fact that *caring* is an integral part of the process. However, there is no widespread consensus as to what the term caring really entails. It was Morse and her colleagues who reported that the five basic conceptualizations, or the basics of caring, can be characterized as follows:

Caring as a human trait

Caring as a moral imperative or an ideal

Caring as an effect

Caring as an interpersonal relationship

Caring as a therapeutic intervention

You will see that the term transpersonal human caring is often associated with Jean Watson's theory and Science of nursing, like the Art and Science of human caring. Watson defined the process of human caring as the moral idea of nursing, in which the relationship between the whole self of the nurse and the whole self of the patient protects the vulnerability and preserves the dignity and humanity of the patient. This emphasis on the *whole self* – the whole of both the nurse and the patient – requires the addition of the word transpersonal in Watson's framework, and in the discussion of human caring as it relates to the practice of holistic nursing.

It is within a transpersonal perspective that you will come to see that people are more than merely the body physical and the mind contained within that body. It is a transpersonal perspective that acknowledges that all people are body, mind, and spirit and that the interaction between people engages with each of these aspects of the self. It is a nurse with a transpersonal perspective who recognizes that this is a fact of human interaction and not an event that is optional. A holistic nurse recognizes, as suggested by Watson, that there is something beyond the personal, separate selves of the nurse and the patient who is involved in the act of caring.

So, what are the basic tenets, then, of transpersonal human care and healing? Let's take a look.

The objectives of the nurse healer in lieu of the transpersonal self

There are different objectives where it comes to holistic healing keeping the transpersonal self in focus.

> The very first thing that one needs to do, is look at what the right relationship would look like if applied to something that you wanted to heal in yourself.

> Then one must think of ways in which one can create their very own healing environment

> One must explore an area of their very own personal woundedness that has healed, and has made them a better nurse in the process.

In a nutshell, transpersonal healing is all about crossing one's limits and boundaries where it comes to their very own egos so that they drop them and focus on what is really important – the person they are taking care of.

When nurses enter into a caring relationship with a patient, bringing with them an acknowledgment and appreciation of the mind, body and spirit dimensions of their very own human existence, it can be safe to say that they are engaged in a transpersonal human healing process.

It is in this type of environment that the nursing professionals know that they are not only interconnected with the patient but with the entire cosmos as well. They know that the ground that they are walking along with the patient is nothing short of being sacred ground and that neither them nor their patients will be the same again after the experience.

Therefore, the transpersonal healing process is such in which the caregiver becomes one with the patient, coming to understand that they might be separate but in essence, they are part of one whole. It is really a higher calling, and one comes to understand this when seen through the eyes of the transpersonal self. It is through this transpersonal healing process that both of them are changed.

The field of consciousness that has been created through the transpersonal process of healing has the ability to heal the patient long after the bond between the patient and the caregiver has expired. In a sense, therefore, it can be termed as timeless. The nurses, too, benefit from this process and this, in turn, helps them provide even better care for their patients. Healing the transpersonal way is extremely energizing and satisfying.

It is often assumed that nurses burn out as a result of caring too much. However, nurses of today are far more likely to burn out for an altogether different reason: the difficulty for finding the time to care for the patient with their whole selves, within the very health care systems that do not value caring.

Chapter 7

The Science and Theory behind Holistic and Human Caring

There is a great deal of science behind what is now commonly known as Holistic Healing. There was a lot of groundwork established by some pioneers in the field, resulting in some theories that formed the framework of this wonderful modern practice.

Let's take a look at the most important ones.

The Theories behind Holistic and Human Caring

The Intersystem Model

The nursing theories of the interactive processes are found philosophically on integrative process models, based on the so-called humanistic philosophy. Based on this theory, *every person is a uniform being which constitutes an energy field in constant interaction with their energy field of the universe*. In a nutshell, this theory looks at every person as a holistic being, one that interacts and adapts to every situation he or she faces.

Callista Roy's Adaptation Model

According to this theory, *a person is a I. In order for that person to face that ever-changing world, he or she would have to use biological, psychological and social mechanisms*. So, according to Roy's model, human behavior represents an adaptation to environmental and organic forces. According to Roy, the very purpose of nursing is to aid the person as he adapts to the occurring changes of his biological needs and self-perception.

Rogers's Theory

Rogers suggested that a person is a *uniform energy system that is in constant reciprocal interaction with the energy system of the universe*. This theory had a drastic effect on the nursing field and encouraged nurses to deal with patients as a whole unit, both during care design and provision. According to Rogers, the nursing environment aims towards providing a harmonious interaction between the person and his or her environment, and also serves to reinforce the cohesion and wholeness of a person's energy field and environment, in order to achieve the highest possible health potential.

Newman's Health Care System Model

According to this theory, *a person is treated as a whole system with individual interlinked parts and subparts*. It proposes that stress factors take their toll on people, who have, however, flexible resistance limits and back-ups that help them defend themselves against these very stress factors. In lieu of this model, you will find that nursing is directed towards recognizing a person's standards in interaction with the environment, and accepting that interaction is an awareness development process.

Parse's Theory

This final theory in the realm of holistic nursing proposes that *the human is considered as a Being, of his own will, who actively participates inside the world*. He suggests that health status is our way of existence inside this world.

The Ethical Theories behind Holistic Nursing

You will find that there are many nurses who will turn away in frustration when asked about the ethical theories that are behind holistic nursing. This is because in the past it has been difficult to correlate these theories with conventional clinical situations. In order to make these theories meaningful, it is important to think of situations in which they might apply to the current clinical practice.

There have been a number of ethical theories that have played an important part in Western civilization, and have laid the foundation for the development of modern ethics. For instance, the *Aristotelian theory* that is based on the individual's manifesting special virtues and developing his or her very own character. Now Aristotle (384 – 322 B.C.) believed that an individual who practices the virtues of temperance, courage, integrity, justice, and honesty, will know almost intuitively what to do in a particular situation or conflict.

Or perhaps we can take into account the system of *Emmanuel Kant* (1724 -1804) who formulated the historical Christian idea of the Golden Rule, 'So act in such a way as your act becomes a Universal for all mankind'. Kant was very concerned with the personhood of human beings, and persons as moral agents.

There are yet other ethical theories that are highly instrumental in understanding the holistic approach to ethics, and these include the *Utilitarianism theory* of Jeremy Bentham and John Stuart Mill and the natural rights theory of John Locke. Briefly put, the utilitarian view of Bentham and Mill proposes that the consequences of our actions are the primary concern, the means justify the end, and every human being has a personal concept of good and bad. On the other hand, the natural rights theory of Locke was the forerunner of the U.S. Declaration of Independence, as it included the tenet that individuals have inalienable rights and that other individuals have an obligation to respect those very rights. There is yet another theory, the *Contractarian theory* of Hobbes that goes on to state that all morality involves a social contract indicating what individuals can and cannot, do.

There is yet another way of viewing ethics, and this is in terms of the two traditional forms: the *deontologic* and the *teleologic.* The former strives to assign duty based on the intrinsic aspects of an act rather than its outcome. Here you will find that action is morally defensible, on account of its intrinsic nature. By contrast, the latter assigns duty or obligation based upon the consequences of the act: here you will find that action is morally defensible based on its *extrinsic nature, or outcome.*

Holistic View of Ethics

It is the holistic view of reality that reopens the vistas of thought that were dominant in the pretechnologic era when people were in fact generally closer to their environment. It is the allure of technology and Science that has led many into being sidetracked into liner and unidirectional thought. Also, while technology has provided conveniences and easy solutions, it has also contributed to a tendency to objectify the universe.

You will find that holistic ethics is a philosophy that couples both the reemerging and rapidly evolving concepts of holism and ethics. In this, there is a basic underlying concept of the integrity and wholeness of all people and of all nature, one that is identified and pursued by finding unity and wholeness within the self and within humanity as well. In the holistic framework, acts are not performed for the sake of the law or for social norms. Rather, they are performed from a desire to do good freely, in order to witness, identify and contribute to the unity of the Self and of the Universe, of which the individual is a part.

While encompassing traditional ethical views, the holistic view is characterized by the Eastern monad in the yin-yang mode and the Western concept of masculine and feminine. It is important to note that holistic ethics is not grounded or judged in the act that is performed, but rather in the conscious evolution of an enlightened individual of raised consciousness, who performs the said act. The primary concern here is the effect of the act on the involved individual and his or her larger self.

Thus, in a nutshell, you will find that holistic ethics are based on some presuppositions like the following.

> There is a Being or Spirit who has actively involved Humanity and the Universe, in whose image we are created.

> There is a divine plan.

> There is purposefulness in the Universe. All occurrences –good or bad, complex or simple – are part of the Divine Plan.

Chapter 8

Healing the Transpersonal Self

We have already touched upon the subject of transpersonal healing and just how effective it can be where it comes to healing patients out there. However, for the very best possible results, one must seek to heal their very own transpersonal selves, before reaching out to heal others. Let's take a look, first, at some of the important questions that nurses must ask themselves when setting out on this journey, with a view to getting only the best results possible.

What do you know about the meaning of healing?

What can you do each day to facilitate healing in yourself?

How can you be an instrument of healing and a nurse healer?

You will find that in the process of healing, the journey is long and fulfilling. There is no dearth of questions, where it comes to understanding the wholeness of human existence.

Let's take a look at a few really important things, when on the path towards healing the transpersonal self.

Things to bear in mind when healing the transpersonal self

Transpersonal healing happens when we help ourselves as well as our families and clients and embrace what is feared most. There should be no denial even in the most extricating of circumstances, in order to allow that healing to happen.

Healing occurs when we seek harmony and balance

Healing is about learning to unlock our highest potential, by opening that which has been closed before.

Transpersonal healing is the fullest expression of ourselves, both light and shadow, as well as the male and female principles that reside within all of us.

Transpersonal healing is all about accessing what we have forgotten about *connections, unity, and interdependence.* When one gets an understanding of the intricate relationship between these three, then healing becomes possible and the experience of the nurse as an instrument of healing becomes actualized.

In transpersonal healing, the nurse healer facilitates another person's growth towards wholeness (of mind, body, and spirit) or assists them with their recovery from an illness or even helps them transition peacefully towards the realm of death.

In transpersonal healing, the focus is on care, love, and compassion (aided with technology where necessary) in order to bring a patient to the prime of their health.

Therefore, you will find that in the process of transpersonal healing, healing takes on an entirely different meaning. It really becomes something that is larger than all of us (and this first begins with the step of one accepting that they are merely a part of the bigger picture itself).

At the very same time, this does not mean that conventional therapy needs to be replaced with transpersonal healing. In fact, transpersonal healing serves as a very nice complement to the process of conventional therapy. The great part about transpersonal healing is the fact that not only does it work (and very well at that, mind you), but it is extremely cost-effective too. All the more reason, then, to place a greater emphasis on it in the workplace.

Chapter 9

The Purpose of Holistic Nursing

Of course, by now we all have a sense of all that holistic nursing entails, and just how effective it can be when treating the individual as a whole. However, it is necessary to delve deeper into the purpose of holistic nursing, with a view to understanding exactly why it is here to stay.

The Purpose of Holistic Nursing

To create an emphasis on wellness, not illness.

This is true. Holism is really about treating the patient as a whole, and thanks to that wonderful philosophy you get treated on all the three levels – physical, mental and spiritual. Therefore, if one might come in to be treated for a physical ailment, he or she might find that at the end of the process they have been healed on more than just the physical level. What is really promoted here, thus, is the wellness of the person on the whole.

To afford the patients a lot more options.

When you are going in for the conventional system of healing, you will find that you are limited to simply *medicines and machines*. However, when you are subject to holistic nursing, you will find that it affords you a lot of wonderful opportunities. There are wonderful therapies that have been proven to work; therapies like reflexology, yoga, and meditation. Along with these wondrous therapies, they can go in for the traditional therapies as well, and the synergistic effect of the two might be just what the doctor ordered, to get them up and about again.

To treat people of all ages.

There are some traditional modes of healing that can only be used for some age groups. Not so in the case of holistic nursing, no. It can be used to help the lives of people of all ages who might be suffering from an ailment of some kind.

To get to the root cause of the problem at hand.

A lot of the patients that come in to be treated have underlying causes that are rooted in things like their poor diet, bad relationships, and increased stress levels. A holistic nurse will get to the root of their problem by seeing exactly what it is that might have caused the problem they have come to get treated. This is important because it not only addresses issues like headaches and backaches in the short term, but it helps resolve them in the long run as well. The emphasis here, as we have already touched upon, is on fixing the problem and not merely treating its symptoms.

To form real relationships.

Where it comes to holistic nursing, you will find that patients not only get into good relations with the wonderful nurses that are treating them, but they are also encouraged to form those very real relationships with themselves. That is one of the key factors that are integral in getting them to see great improvements in their overall well being.

Healing: The Goal of Holistic Nursing

It has become increasingly clear in the last few years, that healing has become the primordial goal of holistic nursing. You will find that while caring might be the context of the very same, the end goal is and will always be healing.

The word heal has its origins in the Anglo-Saxon word Haelan, which means to be or to become whole.

Now, to define what is whole is another matter entirely. What is being whole, really? Does the pursuit of being whole entail working towards an end goal –that of being whole? Or is it perhaps a state of perfection of body, mind, and spirit? Is it a state or a process, and might it be dependent on the functioning and structure of the body? Is it really possible for someone to be not whole?

Is wholeness something that comes and goes, or is it something that one can hold on to? For instance, you might think you are whole today, after having recently been through a holistic nursing treatment, but is this state something that you can hold on to, or is it merely ephemeral? Might you find yourself in a state once again where you feel you are in the doldrums and need that kind of treatment once again?

The good news is holistic treatment ingrains in you all the necessary tools to help sustain your health in the future. That is why, it is possible to hold on to that state of well being, thanks to the holistic nurses who have installed those very tools in you; tools that will help you fight against the devils that have plagued you in the past. There might be some things that you simply can't control, but it can be safe to say that a good deal is in your hands.

In fact, this process of brainstorming should be done by every holistic nurse out there. When they come to discover what it is that makes their very own selves whole, they will have a greater deal of understanding where it comes to treating their patients with a view to making them whole as well. In the end, no single perspective might be exactly the same as the other, but one thing will be common: the healing of the body, mind, and spirit as the end goal.

It is the very process of healing that will make us whole. Many people might feel that they are whole when they are not; just imagine how they would feel if they were really whole? Sometimes, one might just have to go through sickness in order to be healed at all levels. It's ironical, but so many of us are living lives that are not completely whole, yet don't know it at all. Once the process of healing is complete, though, one will come to realize exactly what they have been missing out on in this splendid life and take themselves to the very next level of being altogether.

Healing as the Emergence of Right Relationship

Harmony is defined as an ordered or aesthetically pleasing set of relationships among the elements of the whole.

Wholeness is commonly described as the harmony of body, mind, and spirit.

Therefore, when harmony is put in conjunction with healing, it is essential to know what the aesthetic components of healing are, in addition to the commonly known scientific ways.

There are other synonyms for the word harmony that include *integrity, connection, and unity*. These very words tend to suggest that wholeness is not really a state of any kind, but is, in fact, a process that fundamentally deals with relationships.

Therefore, healing is the emergence of the right relationship at, between or among any levels of the human relationship. It is dynamic and it always affects the whole person, no matter at what level the shift occurs.

The thing is, human beings are systems that are self-organizing and are capable of striving towards order, transcendence, and transformation. The healing process itself is inherent within every person. This urge towards healing and the right effect, when manifested, can be thought of as the *'Haelean effect'*.

In the context of these principles, you will see that the right relationship is not a moral judgment: about discerning what is good and bad or right and wrong. It is, in fact, the way of understanding the quality of patterns and organization. The inherent tendency of any living system is to actualize its deep nature. Therefore, you will find that something as simple as an acorn wanting to be something as magnificent as an acorn tree. What one gets when they are not in the right relationship, is really a tendency towards self-dissolution.

Therefore, the right relationship might be thought of as any point within the system that supports, encourages and allows actualization at any or all levels.

Therefore, with the emergence of the right relationship at any level, body, mind or spirit, you will find that the following result.

> The coherence of the whole body-mind-spirit is increased

> There is decreased disorder in the whole body-mind-spirit

> Free energy is maximized in the whole body-mind-spirit

> Autonomy and choice are maximized in the whole body-mind-spirit

> The capacity for creative unfolding of the whole body-mind-spirit is increased

Sometimes you will find that the right relationship emerges at the spiritual level before it appears anywhere else. Thus, you will find that in moments of deep love and gratitude, people enter into the right relationship with the *One*. It is found that these people have a great capacity to heal.

In a nutshell, holistic nurses egg their patients along the path to self-actualization. The idea is to transform their previous selves and become something higher than they erstwhile were. The goal is not merely on recovery, but on something much greater. This is the growth process of nature.

In the words of Florence Nightingale herself,

'The goal is to put the patient in the best condition so that nature can act on him'.

Healing as a Final Result

It has been well established that the purpose of holism is healing. While we all know what healing is all about, let's take a closer look at the same to gain some valuable insights about the holistic healing process.

When it comes to healing, the same factors that one would have used to establish the process of curing, do not apply. For instance, how can one exactly pinpoint and say that the body-mind-spirit is completely integrated? It might be easy to see if the symptoms and signs of disease of a patient are present or not, but it is entirely another to speculate about the former.

It was *Carper* who outlined the four methods of knowing for nursing: *empiric, aesthetic, ethical and personal.*

Of course, the data that is gathered by the five senses and their extensions through the use of technology is a very important factor in gauging the well being of an individual. However, it is by no means the end way in which one can ascertain if a patient has been completely healed.

To know that healing has happened, we need more than merely the aforementioned empirical knowledge. The very reason that the process of healing is creative and unpredictable, lends credence to the fact that the best way to gauge if healing is really happening or not, would be the subjective knowing of both the patient as well as the nurse.

Most of the nurses out there have had the privilege of attending a moment in which the healing process has occurred. They know that sense of wonder when it arrives, and they know it at an intuitive level. The nurse looks at the patient and the patient looks at the nurse, and they both *just know*. Neither of them might even be able to describe in totality what happened or what brought the shift along, but they simply know that it is *real*.

Sometimes, it is through the aesthetic route that the process of healing happens. You will find the patients who are recovering, literally *draw the shift* from despair to hope or fear to peace. You might even find that things like *music* and *movement* become indicators of a patient's surge in progress.

69

The thing is, none of these indicators of healing can be predicted. There is really no fixed formula to determine exactly how long the hospital stay should be. However, they are the most valid indicators. It is here, really, that holistic nurses have the opportunity to ascertain the wellness of the patient on the whole and not merely look at it as a series of physical outcomes.

Therefore, the outcome of healing is really a combination of all the factors – intuitive, aesthetic and even empirical, that all serve to establish the wellness of the patient in their own unique way. It is definitely subjective, but then that is the very reason you have these wonderful holistic nurses to gauge who is really well, amongst those who aren't.

The Wounded Healer

With a view to gain a deeper perspective into holistic nursing, it is important to realize this one truth in life: *Everyone in this world is wounded.*

Life simply doesn't allow anyone to escape its radar and escape unscathed. Therefore, while it is a matter of fact that being wounded is not optional, what remains optional is what one chooses to do with being wounded. The beautiful part about holistic nursing is it allows nurses to help others and heal them doing the kind of work that their very own woundedness requires. In so doing, what they are really doing is becoming wounded healers for others, in the process.

The wounded healer is certainly not perfect because he or she is done with life's pains and is now healed and whole; rather, the healer is someone who knows well what it means to be wounded and the importance of ongoing healing and caring with a view to promoting wholeness in the patient.

The wounded healer is one who has undertaken the process of healing themselves and is thus a courageous warrior on the path to healing others. He or she is not afraid of the healing journey and can guide others on their path towards healing, and console them the very next moment, when the journey shifts (because it always tends to).

What's even more beautiful about holistic nursing is the fact that holistic nurses know their own limitations. Thus, if a patient is touching them in an area of theirs that is still wounded, they will gracefully pass them on to another holistic nurse who does not need healing in that area, so that they can take care of them in a much more capable manner than they themselves can. So, the patient's care will never be compromised by their ability to provide the best care for them. The more that these nurses become and healed themselves, you will find that their capacity to provide care for their patients also increases. As they grow in self-love, their compassion, and mercy for others increases. It can't be better said than in the words of *Frances Vaughan*, a transpersonal psychologist:

"Healing happens more easily through us when we allow it to happen to us. In this way, the wounded healer who, at the existential level, identifies with the pain and suffering of

those he or she attempts to heal, becomes the healed healer who, being grounded in emptiness and compassion, can facilitate healing more effectively."

As nurses heal more and more themselves, they become increasingly aware of that sacred trust that is granted to them when they have the privilege of taking care of someone else with a view to healing them to the best of their abilities. They accept this very privilege and its demands and responsibilities without so much as batting an eyelid because the wounded healer always wants to give something back to society. In the end, it becomes all about others, not themselves.

Chapter 10

Enhanced Listening

In the pursuit of providing the best holistic care possible, nurses have to focus on what the patient is trying to say and then communicate with them in the best manner possible.

This non-intrusive way of sharing a patient's thoughts and feelings is known as *Enhanced Listening*. To put it in a nutshell, you hear what the patient is saying, repeat that which you have heard, and then check with the patient to make sure that your reflection is correct. What makes enhanced listening different from ordinary listening is the fact that you don't merely *listen to the words*, but rather try to reflect on the feeling or the intent behind the words.

You will find that enhanced listening helps the patients clarify and articulate their inner processes. It can be a most moving experience for a patient when he or she finds a nurse who actually listens to them. This enhanced listening is all the more relevant in a hospital setting, where a lot of patients report themselves as feeling isolated and invisible. Besides building the patient's sense of self, this process of enhanced listening can actually be most rewarding for the nurse, too.

There is one very useful tool that can help patients where it comes to getting a real change to unfold in their lives. It is called *focusing*. In the famous words of the great Antoine de Saint Exupery,

"It is only with the heart that one can see rightly; what is essential is invisible to the eye." -The Little Prince

Focusing is based on the very notion that the body and the mind are intimately connected. For instance, when you have *'butterflies in your stomach'* before a performance review, you most certainly know what that means, don't you?

When people are ill or simply undergoing stress, what happens is they become absorbed by their bodies and symptoms like pain and anxiety claim all their attention. That's where focusing steps in. It encourages one to connect in an emphatic manner with his or her body, and try to understand the psychological implications of the bodily sensations they are experiencing, without in any way getting overwhelmed.

This sense of focusing can be used very well by holistic nurses who want to help their patients heal well. They can tell them to focus on what they are feeling in a friendly manner, and not merely try and resist it or shake it off. In so doing, they might actually help the patients come to some startling conclusions about how they are really feeling, and thus help them realize that what they were stressing over, was not all that stressful at all.

This kind of enhanced listening will allow the patient to get distance from their pain and perhaps even befriend it. They can help them sense how their body would be without that very pain, and help them work compassionately with the feelings that are accompanying that very pain – feelings of anger, disappointment or helplessness.

Part 3

Holistic Nursing Research and Studies

In order to gain a deeper sense of awareness into how the process of healing actually works, it's interesting to take a ride into the psychophysiology of healing the body and mind, in order to gain a deeper perspective of the healing dynamics.

Chapter 11

Psychophysiology of Healing the Body and Mind

Where it comes to the psychophysiology of healing the body and mind, a lot of interesting things are brought into the light. Let's have a look at some of the nurse healer objectives where it comes to this valuable subject, in order to gain some valuable insights.

Theoretical

The holistic nurse needs to articulate a comprehensive conceptual model of body-mind interactions. He or she needs to interpret the application of selected models, theories and research in the field of psychoneuroimmunology. Furthermore, there is a need to explain the interconnections of mind modulation, and the autonomic, endocrine, immune and neuropeptide systems.

Clinical

As far as the clinical objectives are concerned, the nurse must strive to recognize the implications of body-mind interactions as far as clinical practice is concerned. The knowledge of body-mind interactions must be incorporated in the process of planning nursing interventions.

Personal

One's own patterns of body-mind interactions as expressed in attitudes, tensions, and images, must be identified. Furthermore, the implications of one's own body patterns for self-care and self-healing must be recognized.

Bell's theorem

According to Bell's theorem, *the whole determines the action of the parts, and changes occur instantaneously.* Experience would serve to teach us that not all people respond to the same treatment in the same way. For instance, in the case of peptic ulcers, the *Sippy diet* worked wonders for some while it didn't work at all for others. Did those that recovered, recover because of the synergistic effect of diet and rest, or was there some other intervening factor that led to their recovery? It could be that for some patients, the imposed rest actually increased their stress and the restrictive diet only served to exacerbate their ulcer.

What one can take away from this is that there is no ordered sequence for things to take place. Healing does not take time, but rather is dependent on the hope and belief that transcend time. *Belief, thoughts, and feelings* are all important parts of the configuration, and as such, each has a great role to play where it comes to the patient being healed.

Personality and Wellness

There have been researchers in the past, who have unsuccessfully tried to link illness with certain personality traits. For instance, taking the very example of peptic ulcers in consideration, it is found that persons with peptic ulcers do not have any more personality conflagrations than the general public that doesn't have those peptic ulcers.

However, there are several researchers who have found that there are indeed personality traits that are associated with illness. For instance, *Schwartz* found that people who attend to symptoms, sensations, and feelings, those that connect those signals to events in their lives and who express what is happening have a stronger immune profile and a healthier cardiovascular system than those who do not. This capacity grew on to become the ACE (Attend, Connect, Express) factor.

Information Theory

According to Damasio, our emotions and feelings are sources of vital information. The emotions are in fact life-regulating phenomena that help maintain our health by making adaptive changes in our body states and form the basis for feelings. The information that is generated by these processes is designed to be protective, and more complex than reflexes.

The Santiago Theory of Cognition

In this theory based on cognition, even the cells that make up the immune system perceive their environment and will, for example, move to the site of a wound and increase in numbers to deal with an invading organism. Despite the absence of a brain, you will find that cognition is present. In fact, in this event, it can be perceived as 'embodied action'. Perception and action in these cells are really inseparable. Furthermore, it is seen that a living organism chooses which stimuli from the environment will trigger structural changes. Also, not all changes in an organism are acts of cognition. For instance, a person that is injured in let's say, a car accident, does not specify or even direct those structural changes. However, the other structural changes like perception and response of the circulatory system that accompany the imposed changes, are acts of cognition.

The Santiago theory helps to explain how human beings receive, generate and transduce information. The new ideas and events call for changes in the bodymind – the neural pathways and consciousness team up to enable information transduction.

In layman terms, a person who has severe asthma attacks might become despondent on recalling that their own mother struggled with that very disease, which only got worse as she grew older. This is when the holistic nurse might intervene, and teach the patient to monitor her asthma with the help of a flow meter. In time the client will be able to see a pattern to her attacks and be able to identify potential triggers. She will gain a newfound understanding of body-mind connections and use both traditional and holistic interventions in order to disrupt those triggers. These results will result in a change in the pattern of attacks of that patient, and they will diminish in frequency and severity.

Emotions and the Neural Tripwire

According to the traditional view in neuroscience, the sensory organs transmit signals to the thalamus and from there to the sensory process areas of the neocortex, which translates the symbols into perceptions and attaches meanings. The signals then move the limbic system, which sends the appropriate response to the body.

All that has changed now, with the discovery of a separate, smaller bundle of neurons leading directly from the thalamus to the amygdala. Sensory impulses go directly from the sensory organs to the amygdala, thus allowing for a faster response. The amygdala triggers an emotional response even before the person in whom it is triggered, begins to know what is happening.

The amygdala sends impulses through the brain and to the body. In case the experience is a traumatic one, the amygdala will respond with extra strength. Now what happens is that key changes take place in the locus ceruleus, which is responsible for the regulation of catecholamines. In the process, adrenaline and noradrenaline are released.

After this, other limbic structures like the hippocampus and the hypothalamus respond, and the typical body responses like *fight or flight or faint or freeze*, are brought about by the main stress hormones. The person is prepared to meet the danger thanks to the changes in the brain's opioid system, which allows for the release of endorphins.

New Scientific Understanding of Living Systems

Recent developments in Science show human beings in an entirely different light. Gone are the days when people would look at the world in mechanistic fashion; like through the lenses of *Descartes* and perhaps even *Newton*. Now, all that has given way to a holistic and even ecological, view. You will come to see that the commonly used term bodymind includes the body, mind, and spirit as a whole. In the 1920s there were discoveries in Quantum Physics that shocked the entire world. Heisenberg described the world as *'A complicated tissue of events, in which connections of different kinds alternate, overlap or combine, and therefore define the texture as a whole.'*

In the past, the properties of the parts were used to describe the whole. Now, the converse was also true: the whole also determined the properties of the parts. This was all thanks to the advances in quantum physics.

When we take a closer look at the body, you will come to see that all its parts work together. Health and disease are really *indivisible*; both of them are natural and necessary. For instance, fever might be seen as a sign of illness, but it is also perceived as a sign of the body's healthy response to a threat. What fever does, really, is indicate that the hypothalamic set point of the body has changed. This kind of alteration occurs in the presence of pyrogens like bacteria and viruses. Fever can actually be beneficial because it helps to defend the body against the very pyrogens that are attacking it. That is why, using medications to lower fever, especially in the first 24 hours, might actually serve to interfere with this very important defense mechanism of the body.

It is largely on account of the *Systems Theory*, that human beings and their environments make up an interconnected dynamic system in which a change at any point might affect changes at other points. The idea that the world is hierarchical, with each level being organized separately, has now been replaced with a new understanding of relatedness and context. A dysfunction in any one system of the body will echo through the others. For instance, a dysfunction of the endocrine system, i.e. hypothyroidism, might manifest itself in thinning hair or perhaps even clinical depression. Changes in one system result in changes in another system and a system might even initiate changes in itself, much as the pituitary gland will increase its secretion of TSH (Thyroid Stimulating Hormone).

It has thus been seen that no longer can scientists describe their work as being the ultimate missing part of a jigsaw puzzle of some kind. You will come to see that all the things and events happening in one's life are really connected and relative within the whole. The thoughts, feelings, and actions that one's life is comprised of, actually serve to influence a person's state of health and illness.

The Quantum Theory

In the 1920s, there were discoveries in quantum physics that shocked the entire scientific community. It was seen that the old way of viewing the phenomena, no longer fit. It was *Heisenberg* who described the changed world as '*a complicated tissue of events, in which connections of different kinds alternate, overlap or combine and thereby determine the texture as a whole*'. Whereas in the past the properties and behaviors were seen as determining those of the whole, the advances in quantum physics shed light on the fact that the converse was true as well: that the whole also defined the behavior of the parts.

It was the very realization that systems are integrated wholes that cannot be understood simply by analysis that shattered the scientific certitude. No longer was it possible to believe that all questions would have answers, no matter how much time and money was invested in them. Instead, there was a fundamental shift towards accepting that all scientific theories have their limitations.

In fact, the scientific explanation, rather than providing concrete answers, gives way to the emergence of yet more questions. Even one piece of data can change the entire way we see things.

Also, scientific findings demonstrate a world that is changing. It was *Planck* who found out that radiant energy was emitted from light sources in discrete amounts or 'quanta', and that the changes in the amount of radiant energy occurred in leaps and not sequential steps. It was *Bohr* who extended Planck's discovery to the field of subatomic particles and proposed that electrons could move from one orbit of energy to another. It is seen that the behavior of light does not follow one fixed set of rules. It possesses the qualities of both *waves* as well as *particles.* It must be noted, though, that it's not as though one explanation is right and the other is wrong. Rather, they are both useful in demonstrating the behavior of light in different situations.

You will come to see that the world is complex and unified. There are parts that complement each other and also participate in the whole. In the very same fashion, all parts of the body work together.

The Theory of Relativity

It was early in the twentieth century that *Einstein* developed a system of mechanics that acknowledges the relative character of motion, velocity, and mass, as well as the interdependence of matter, time and space. The theory of relativity is based on the principle that there is no absolute frame of reference that is independent of the observer. You will see that each person views the other via his or her very own perspective (and this includes his or her personal biases, as well). Einstein characterized the nature of this revelation dawning on him, as having the ground pulled out from under him.

It is seen that even religious beliefs have a great impact on health, although it is not quite understood how. It was *Koenig and associates* who reported that Christian people who attend religious services at least once a week, and who read the Bible and pray regularly, have consistently lower diastolic blood pressure readings than those who don't. It is this lower diastolic pressure, one that is an indicator of when the heart relaxes, which is an important indicator of sound health. Now, it is not clearly known if the religious activities of these people influence the blood pressure, or if there is a spiritual orientation that accompanies these activities that makes the difference, but the fact remains: *the difference is there.*

There are studies that have used imaging devices that have shown that mindfulness meditation serves to strengthen the neurological circuits that calm a part of the brain that acts as a trigger for fear and anger. Furthermore, the studies using encephalographs found that the brains of the people who practiced mindfulness increased the amount of activity in the brain that is associated with positive emotions. Happiness and inner balance are indeed crucial where it comes to survival. After the events that rocked the United States of America on September 11, 2001, it was evident that modern technology when coupled with hatred, can lead to great suffering. Therefore, it becomes imperative that we cultivate our inner development if we are to keep those emotions of ours in check.

Principles of Self-Organization

In the past, living systems were viewed from two perspectives: in terms of structure (physical matter) and pattern (the configuration of relationships). Whereas structure is concerned with quantities – things weighed and measured, patterns are expressed by a map of the configuration of relationships and are concerned with qualities. There are qualities, like color or size that were once considered accidental characteristics. For instance, a bike might be green or perhaps even red in color. It might have a light or a heavy frame, and it remains a bicycle as long as it has the configuration of relationships that are consistent with a bicycle.

You will come to see that systems, whether they are living or nonliving, are nothing short of being configurations of ordered relationships whose attributes are the properties of pattern. The bicycle, that is a nonliving system, is comprised of a number of components that are arranged to perform a particular function. The various kinds of bicycles, like mountain bicycles and touring bicycles, embody the essential characteristics that comprise a bicycle. In a nutshell, bicycles have a structure with specific components and they operate as bicycles as long as the patterns of structure that define them as bicycles, remains.

Living systems, on the other hand, are fundamentally different from nonliving systems. They do not function

88

mechanically and are not explained merely by physical principles. You will come to see that the components of living systems are interconnected by internal feedback loops in a nonlinear fashion, and are capable of self-organization.

The activity of living systems is not only purposeful but also seems to be under the direction of an overall design or purpose. You will come to see that the pattern of organization of living systems includes a fundamental, self-organizing force that is known as autopoiesis. Even then, if the pattern of a living system is destroyed then the living system dies, even though all the components of the system are intact. You will come to see that the living system cannot be restored simply by recreating the pattern. On the other hand, a nonliving system, like the instance of the bicycle that we have touched upon above, will regain its functionality once its parts are reassembled.

It has come to be seen that living systems do not rest in a steady state of balance as their nonliving counterparts do. In fact, they operate far from equilibrium. You will see that the stability in living systems embodies change. The relationships are not linear, but rather extend in all directions. The process of bifurcation occurs and generates new feedback loops. So, living systems regulate and recreate themselves.

Cognition (Life Process) is the link between pattern and structure in a living system. You will find that Life Process is really tantamount to being 'the activity involved in the continual embodiment of the system's pattern of organization'. It is related to the process of autopoiesis. All

89

living systems are cognitive systems, and cognition actually serves to indicate the existence of an autopoietic network. Here you will find that *Structure, Pattern, and Process* are inextricably linked, in a living system.

The thing is, organisms do not merely function mechanically. In fact, they are under the direction of an overall design or purpose. Let's take in consideration here the symptoms that are experienced by patients, which represent attempts to regain health, and are therefore signals of stability and not of breakdown. It is none other than the human immune system that recognizes an invading organism as dangerous, and in turn, quickly reacts to counter the threat. You will see that symptoms are really signs of the inherent organization and adaptability of a living system and one cannot afford to mistakenly predict the outcome of these complex relationships between organisms. While one person might become sick and perhaps even die, another might be unaffected and yet infect others who come into contact with him or her. You will see here that even the invading organisms, that are also living systems, learn and adapt. It is the very ability of pathogens to modify themselves and develop resistance to antibiotics, which is a striking example of a living system's ability to reorganize.

Identity and Wellness

We all think we know exactly who we are, but how much of that is really true? You will find that whilst on the path to holistic wellness, a lot of things will come to light that you might not have erstwhile been prepared for. These are things that will indeed shake your vision of the way you see things and might make you see the world in an entirely different light.

Some of the things that you will come to experience with your sense of identity whilst on the path to wellness are as follows:

You will lose that sense of comfort. Been stuck in that comfort zone for long? Well, ever imagine how wonderful it might be if you stepped out of that very space? On the path towards holistic healing, you will find that you lose that sense of connection that you erstwhile had with certain things, places and behaviors. This might come as a rude shock to the system, but don't worry (and now you certainly don't need to because you have been warned in advance). This is nothing short of being a normal transition in the process of waking up and uncovering your real identity.

You will feel lonely. You might come to experience an increasing sense of alienation and feel extremely lonely when you are going through these holistic wellness changes in your life. This stems from the fact that you might feel that you are the only one going through something like this. However, you should give yourself a pat on the back for undergoing such a radical transition – one that will ultimately lead you to being more connected with the environment and people around you, in a way like no other.

You might have feelings of regret. Of course, you might think that this wonderful transition that you are undergoing, should have happened a lot sooner in your life. This might only serve to make you look back in regret, and that only means that you won't be aiding your progress in any way. Rather than looking back, look ahead at the wonderful life in front of you.

You will see the negativity amidst the positivity. As you begin to see the wonderful effects that newfound sense of positivity is having in your life, there might be thoughts of negativity that stem to the forefront too, on account of you being increasingly aware of the things around you. What you need to do, is to not let that negativity affect you in any which way. Instead, direct your attention to the positive things – the ones that will take your life to that next level.

It's really not all that easy when you are grappling with that sense of identity whilst on the path towards holistic healing. However, one thing will be clear in the end: you will come to see yourself for who you truly are, having skinned away those fake layers that have been part of you so long.

State-Dependent Memory and Recall

The thing is, what people remember depends largely on their mood and feelings at the very time of their experience. Feelings are integral to the human experience; not merely an extravagance. You will find that the *ligands*, which are the emotion-carrying molecules, bind to the cellular receptors and send a message to the cell where they can be stored as memories.

Feelings and actions are really intertwined. You might have already come to see that people are more likely to help others when they are in a good mood, and conversely, they might be more likely to hurt others when they are in a bad mood. In much the same way, feelings and memories are also intertwined. You will come to see that the thoughts that occur to us through our daily routines are really nothing short of being repeated patterns of erstwhile memories and their associative emotional connections.

You will come to see that memories come hand-in-hand with emotions that are in turn influenced and affected by the context in which they are acquired. For instance, a memory that is particularly traumatic in nature will be stamped harder in one's memory than most others. Now, stimuli in new situations can attach to and reawaken those past memories. You will come to see that these reactivated thoughts and emotions serve to direct our thoughts and actions in the present.

Feelings can play a major role in the healing of the bodymind. There has been recent work that has been done with patients suffering from PTSD (Post-Traumatic Stress Disorder) that has revealed that relearning is the route to healing. *Writing therapy, art therapy and traditional talk therapies* are ways in which the pictures that are frozen in the amygdala can be unfrozen. At the very same time, there is interesting body work that is also being used to unfreeze pockets of energy frozen in the body.

The thing is because people have network responses with the systems that they contain, the process of healing can occur in several directions.

The recent discoveries in Science have led to a lot of interesting discoveries as compared with the old ones.

> Memories are not really stored in any specific part of the brain, as was thought earlier. Rather, they are stored in multiple overlapping areas. They can be retrieved entirely by a stimulus to more than one area of the brain. The loss of any single chunk of memory can be attributed more to the amount of brain damage than towards a specific site of injury.

> The ability to retrieve what was lost when the brain was injured by a gunshot wound or perhaps even a cardiovascular stroke often returns, although the regeneration of neurons is not possible (as it was thought to be earlier).

> Paranormal healing, which is healing that is done in metaphysical ways, involves the communication of information in ways that do not conform to the current understanding of receiving, sending and processing energy.

Response to Pain

It is interesting to note the schematics of pain where it comes to holistic healing. Pain can have a great amount of influence where it comes to the outcome of the holistic healing process.

For instance, the phenomenon of the placebo is a paradox of sorts, where it comes to pain. You will come to see that the more pain a person has, the more dramatic it will be his or her reaction to placebo medication.

Certain stimuli like circadian rhythms, the environment, and emotional and physical stressors influence the secretion of hypothalamic hormones. The opioids like enkephalins and endorphins are synthesized in the pituitary and in other parts of the CNS (Central Nervous System). These have morphine-like effects with the receptors throughout the body. In fact, these are the very hormones that produce the commonly experienced 'runner's high'. What they serve to do is to increase a person's pain threshold, and also explain how people can ignore their own severe injuries to save a loved one.

Pain is a universal and multidimensional experience. As a stressor, pain stimulates the very same physiological responses as the other stressors that affect the nervous, endocrine and immune systems. Furthermore, pain memories produce the same psychologic and spiritual outcomes. Just like stress is designed to meet demands, pain is designed to alert people to problems. In fact, it is the significance of the pain that one is experiencing, that shapes the experience itself. The more threatening the diagnosis is, the more intense the level of suffering. For instance, a woman who finds a lump in her breast might suspect that she has cancer. Now, this leads to her facing uncertainty, fear, and pain throughout her diagnosis and treatment. Furthermore, any new pains that might emerge thereafter are interpreted as the return of cancer, therein stimulating psychophysiological responses.

In this case, you will find that talking to the patient concerned, and especially listening to them, might not only serve to reduce the pain but also to help the patient tap into his or her very own personal resources.

Let's now take a look at the two intrinsic types of pain: chronic and acute.

Chronic pain differs from acute pain in the fact that it is prolonged and lasts longer than anticipated based on the etiology of the pain. Prolonged chronic pain might even increase to the point where it becomes the very disease or condition itself. When this happens, there are lifestyle changes that are inevitable, and that often leads to the patients getting depressed and irritable. The good news, however, is that these very chronic pain patterns can be reversed through the aid of nonpharmacologic holistic interventions like *cognitive restructuring, biofeedback, and mental imagery.*

Acute pain, on the other hand, is time-limited, because it occurs with a problem that is identifiable; one that usually responds to diagnosis and treatment. Surgery, injury, and trauma are common reasons for acute pain. You will find here that the healing of tissue damage usually serves to reverse the pain.

Chapter 12

Health and Spirituality

Every human experience has components that are embedded in all three layers – body, mind, and spirit. In the context of spirituality and healing, it is important to remember that the words *healing, whole and holy* actually derive their meaning from the same root: the old *Saxon Hal*, meaning whole.

In accordance with the same, it would be wise to suggest that healing is a spiritual process that by its very nature attends to the wholeness of a person. The process of healing requires the knowledge of the spiritual dimension of the person as well as the healer. Furthermore, there is the knowledge that spirituality permeates every encounter.

This shared relationship serves to acknowledge the common humanity and connectedness between the caregiver and the receiver, and this is something that is basic to healing and is a very manifestation of spirituality.

Let us look at some of the integral things that are related to spirituality where it comes to the promotion of the overall well being of a person.

Mystery

Mystery is something that is inherent to human experience and can be described as a truth that is beyond understanding and explanation. There are many experiences in life that prompt us to ask questions like Why and What if, and it is these very questions that form the core of mystery. You will come to see that spirituality helps where it comes to the seeking of those very questions. It helps people to embrace both the darkness and the light, and appreciate the challenges and gifts of both.

Love

Love is indeed the very essence of life, and it prompts each person to live from the heart, which is the very center from which the ego is detached. Love transcends space and time, and it enables its energy to be shared for healing at many levels. Love is both personal and universal and is a key component of spiritual care.

Suffering

Suffering is one of the core mysteries of life, something people have grappled to understand over time. For some, suffering leads them to undergo a spiritual transformation. For others, suffering leads them to harboring a feeling of hopelessness. Nurses need to discern whether honoring a person's suffering requires action, presence, absence, or perhaps a combination of them all. The ability to be with another person when their suffering has gone beyond help is crucial.

Hope

Hope goes beyond merely wishing or believing. The saying, 'Hope Springs Eternal', reflects the indomitable nature of the spirit and gives way to the realization that tomorrow things might be different from what they are today. Hope helps people to deal with fear and uncertainty and is thus integral to the holistic healing process.

Forgiveness

Forgiveness is also an integral part of the self-healing process, and it is important to note that this is something that one does for themselves, not for others, even though in essence it is the act of extending love and compassion to others.

Chapter 13

Holistic Nursing and Spirituality

When it comes to spirituality in holistic nursing, it is important to note that the process of nurturing the human spirit is really far more important than one might think, where it comes to bringing around the well being of the patient.

Let us first take a look at the objectives of the holistic nurse, where it comes to the realm of spirituality.

Theoretical

Here the goal of the holistic nurse would be to first and foremost describe spirituality and compare and contrast spirituality and religion, in order to understand the very tangible difference between the two. They need to discuss the common elements of spirituality and their various manifestations in different people. They also need to recognize mystery, suffering, hope, and love as spiritual issues, and discuss the interplay of spirituality and psychology.

Clinical

As far as the clinical aspects of spirituality are concerned, one needs to firstly explore the efficacy and place of prayer in healing. They need to discuss listening as an intentional presence and incorporate the different approaches to spiritual assessment into holistic care. Also, they need to describe tangible approaches for responding to spiritual concerns.

Personal

Here, one needs to explore the need for nurses to nurture their own spirits, and the ways in which to do the same. Furthermore, they need to discuss the ways in which ritual, rest and leisure relate to spirituality, and explore ways of naming and nurturing important connections.

Now, let's take a look at the essence of both spirituality and religion so that we can understand the essential difference between the two.

Spirituality

Spirituality is the very essence of our being. It permeates our living in relationships and also serves to infuse our unfolding awareness of who and what we are, our purpose in being and our valuable inner resources. You will come to see that spirituality is active and expressive, and it shapes as well as is shaped by, our life journey. It informs the ways that we live and experience life, the ways in which we encounter mystery and also the ways in which we relate to all aspects of life. It is inherent in the human condition and is expressed and experienced through our connectedness with the Sacred Source, the Self, and Nature.

Religion

Religion, on the other hand, refers to the organized system of beliefs regarding the cause, purpose, and nature of the Universe that is shared by a group of people, and the practices, behaviors and rituals associated with that very system. You will find that religion connects people with shared values, beliefs and practices. In the process it makes clear particular belief systems that are different from other belief systems, thus serving to define the differences between different groups of persons.

Now that we have seen the basic difference between spirituality and religion and understood what spirituality is in essence, let's take a further look at spirituality in greater detail.

Nurturing the Spirit

The spiritual path is a *life path*, and the way that nurses care for themselves has a profound impact on the way they treat others. The attentiveness that they pay to their very own spirit is a key component of integrating spirituality into clinical practice.

Caring for their very own spirit or soul implies that nurses have to take time off for pausing and reflecting on what is happening in their very own lives. They need to see what is happening within and around them, and to take time out for themselves and the relationships that they might be in. In short, they have to be mindful of nourishing their very own spirits.

The very ways that nurses nurture their spirits, will be the ways in which they will nurture the spirits of the people they have been entrusted to take care of. The care of the spirit is indeed a professional nursing responsibility and forms an intrinsic part of holistic nursing. You will find that within a holistic framework, providing spiritual care is nothing short of being an ethical practice - one that will serve to provide dignity to the patients that are being treated – the dignity that they rightfully deserve.

Nurses thus should become competent and confident with spiritual caregiving, and thereby expand their skills where it comes to assessing the spiritual domain. They need to develop and implement the appropriate interventions as well. For instance, one particular barrier where it comes to implementing spirituality into the nursing practice would be the imposition of one's religious beliefs onto another.

The nurses who integrate spirituality into their holistic treatment of others, need to realize that even though the foundation for all that they do might be deeply ingrained in a spiritual belief, acting from this very foundation is certainly not the same as imposing these beliefs and values onto others. In fact, there are many practitioners that believe that the more grounded they are in their very own spiritual practice, the less likely they are to impose their beliefs on others.

All said and done, the attempts to quantify spirituality, even with scales that are more broadly applicable, must be viewed with caution, regarding the results and the effects of such instruments on care. Although quantification might more readily capture the attention of the scientific and the medical communities, the reliance on quantitative measurements might promote the use of diagnostic reasoning and structured interview formats as a substitute for listening.

The goal of holistic healing is to know a person in their fullness, and by focusing on their spiritual component in addition to their bodies and minds, one can be sure of achieving just that in the process.

Using Story and Metaphor in Physical Care

The act of recognizing all persons, including themselves, as ongoing and unfolding stories offers nurses a valuable perspective from which to approach spiritual caregiving. The thing is, spirituality is multidimensional – it reflects the depth and the complexity of a person's being, and embraces that very person's connections with the Sacred Source, the earth, other persons and even the Self.

Story and metaphor often go on to provide a language and form with a view to convey the richness of one's spirituality, when factual statements of experience fail to do so. Stories entertain people and teach them to solve problems. They help them to form identities and are indeed wondrous teachers. There are very few things in this world that can help a person understand something better than a story can.

It is through the art of telling a story that people can learn to know each other from many different perspectives. These stories reveal the experience of emotions, struggles, and relationships that are personal and universal at the very same time. Holistic nurses, in fact, become a part of the story of a patient for that difficult time in their lives. The nurses themselves have been a part of a story; a story that has helped define them and shape them into what they are today. It is the understanding of their very own stories that help them deepen the awareness with which they listen to another person's story.

Therefore, it is absolutely imperative that nurses listen to other people's stories, and even encourage them to tell the same. This exercise can be instrumental in the assessment and intervention in spiritual care. It is these very stories that make it possible to move beyond physical symptoms and diagnoses that are common for a wide variety of patients. It helps one understand that people are not intrinsically the same, even though their ailments might be. The attentiveness to the patient's story thus affords the nurses a unique glimpse into the wholeness and the uniqueness of each patient.

Furthermore, story and metaphor provide a valuable sense of insight into spiritual concerns like supportive or disruptive relationships, questions of meaning or purpose and issues of forgiveness and hope. Listening to stories helps serve as a valuable reminder that at no point is the story of a person finished; rather, it is ongoing.

This sharing of the story and metaphor can also be a valuable nursing intervention. You will find that when they are sharing their stories with a listener who is completely attentive, patients will come to see that they are able to hear their own stories with a newfound sense of appreciation for their own lives. They can share their fears and hopes in a safe space, and in this process, they come to see themselves more clearly and accept themselves in their full humanity. This serves to lead them to participate in the present moment far more consciously.

Holistic Caring Process Considerations

The process of spiritual caregiving requires an understanding of the holistic caring process that is integrative, one in which assessment and intervention might very well be the same process, and where description might be more useful than labeling. The identification of needs in the realm of spirituality does not necessarily go on to indicate impairment or pathology.

The research on spirituality and health leads us to highlight the importance of describing the human spirit in the experience of individual beings. Every person has a story to tell, as we have already touched upon, and it is this story that needs to be understood with the view to providing the best individualistic care. This also means that each person's individual values need to be explored, in order to help us understand what makes them tick.

The evolving nursing diagnoses regarding spirituality are used appropriately by nurses who understand that where it comes to any health concern whatsoever, spirituality is of paramount importance and can simply not be neglected. What is important is that the nurses enter into a kind of collaboration with the patients and their families. They need to determine the appropriate outcomes, develop a plan and organize the overall care in order to incorporate each patient's worldview, values, and selfhood.

You will find that nurses facilitate this well when they promote an atmosphere that is understanding of the spiritual needs of the patient – one that accepts the spiritual experience in its varied forms. The understanding and the awareness of their very own spiritual perspective improve the ability of the nurses to be alert to its influence on their relationships and work. They are able to understand their very own discomfort with a client's spiritual perspective and involve others in order to provide the much-needed care for the client.

The care of the human spirit, which is a fundamental aspect of holistic nursing care, takes place in the context of the significant connections in the person's life. For a time, the nurse enters the client's world, and through the intentional foray into this relationship, she might precipitate the much-needed healing.

Thus, the processes of assessment, planning, diagnosis, and intervening are all experienced within a unique relationship. It is the very recognition that all persons are spiritual beings that leads to the formation of the basis for being alert to the many ways in which people express their spirituality.

It is not merely the simple hearing and validation of the human spirit that is a part of the assessment, but it becomes an important part of the intervention as well. Simply giving patients the opportunity to discuss spiritual concerns enables them to become more spiritually aware.

Forming spiritual connections with one or more colleagues at the workplace can be highly beneficial in the process of helping nurses maintain their spirits in the midst of increasing daily demands. Through the use of awareness and creativity, holistic nurses can use simply any given activity out there, as a way to foster spiritual presence.

Praying and Meditating

You will find that in many traditions, cultural as well as religious, prayer and meditation are spiritual disciplines that are practiced. The holistic nurse, through the virtues of respect and sincerity, can help the patients remember or explore the ways they reach out to God, by appreciating the personal nature of these very disciplines.

The processes of recalling the place and meaning of prayer, and the ways in which they experience the communion with God or the Sacred Source, provides patients with a highly valuable resource. You will find that in the clinical setting, the role of prayer will be determined by both the nurse's and patient's understanding of the same. Clarifying both the need and understanding of prayer is indeed a most valuable aspect of holistic care.

Of course, the nature of all patients is not the same. You will find that while some patients prefer to pray on their very own, yet others want someone else to pray with them or even for them. There are some patients who don't even believe in prayer. The nurses, thus, should be respectful of each person's requests for prayer, be it getting others to pray with them or perhaps even praying for them themselves. It is indeed an important aspect of caring for the spirit when the nurse facilitates the appreciation and practice of prayer in the patient's life.

Where it comes to the process of prayer, imagery can play a really big role in aiding the same. You will come to see that patients who have been cooped up for too long in hospital beds, find it far easier to pray when they can be magically transported through their minds to some other place, like perhaps the ocean or even some sacred temple somewhere. Here it must be noted that family and friends can play a great role when it comes to aiding the patient in the role of using imagery effectively.

Also, assisting the patients to consider the value of rest and leisure in their lives, is an integral part of holistic nursing. You will come to see that the way the nurses take stock of the ways in which they incorporate rest and leisure into their very own lives, is an important component of self-care for them as well. It is all the more important to give rest and leisure some important consideration in today's world, where the norm is simply to fill up every moment in the day so that one can be more productive. The good news is, if you incorporate more rest and leisure into your life, you will find that in the process you become more productive as well.

The role of the holistic nurse is to enhance the patient's conscious awareness of how rest and leisure are, or are not, a part of their lives. Things like regular exercise, music, and imagery are all excellent ways in which one can promote their rest and leisure.

Part 4

Nursing with the Chakras – Energetic Healing

In this section, you will learn all about the wonderful use of chakras, where it comes to the process of healing. Let's take a look!

Chapter 14

Energetic Healing through Holistic Nursing

Energetic healing in its primordial essence is a term that is used to describe healing that alters the subtle flow of energy within or around a person.

When the process of holistic nursing is combined with energetic healing, you will find that there is scope for healing that is life-changing in nature. Holistic nurses use energetic healing to heal a patient of his or her physical, mental or emotional wounds. You will find that pain relief and decreased depression and anxiety are merely a few of the many benefits that are associated with the wondrous process of energetic healing.

Energetic healing can help one grow open to a conscious aspect of their self that is not limited to their physical body or to their emotions and thoughts. *Assagioli* called this the *Higher Self* or *Transpersonal Self*.

The expert healers understand the energetic processes and the structures, including the chakras, meridians, and even auras, and they know exactly when to use the energetic healing approach. Here we are concerned with the use of chakras, so let's probe the same in greater detail.

So, what are chakras, really?

Traditional Explanations of Chakras

In Sanskrit, Chakra means vortex or wheel of light.

There is a great deal of lore about Chakras, but there are two things that are common with all theories:

Chakras exist within and around the body

Chakras are ports for energy exchange with the environment

You will find that chakras bring in energy, give meaning to information and release energy and information. It is through these very chakras that people broadcast their emotions and thoughts before they even speak them. Most traditions identify 7 major chakras that are all located near large collections of nerves or neuroendocrine glands and attribute to them various colors and sounds. A very famous model assigns to them the colors of the rainbow and the tones of an octave. For instance, the root chakra is seen as the color red and heard as the note middle C.

You will see that people stimulate their chakras by the colors they wear and the music they hear. In Physics we have learned that cellular biology is based on minute bundles of energy. It might very well be that chakras bring in those bundles of energy that are transported rapidly through the body by the nervous system and more slowly, but surely, by the meridians.

Let us first take a look at the seven major chakras and what they are associated with.

The Root Chakra: Survival and security

The Second Chakra: Sexuality, sensuality and your passions

The Third Chakra: Emotions

The Fourth Chakra (heart): The love of Self and Others

The Fifth Chakra (throat): Speaking one's own truth about security, creativity and all that they love

The Sixth Chakra (brow): The third eye - Intuition and Perception. This one provides an insight into the activity of the first four chakras

The Seventh Chakra (crown): The Gateway to the Spiritual Realm, to one's higher chakras and their transpersonal self.

So, what makes those chakras really tick? Well, let's take a look at some of the explanations for what makes them work.

The Scientific Explanation of Chakras

Valerie Hunt, a professor of physical therapy at UCLA (The University of California, Los Angeles), obtained actual objective evidence of the activity of chakras. She placed EMG electrodes on the skin of the chakra areas. What she found next was fascinating.

Valerie Hunt found regular, high frequency, wavelike electrical signals that were ranging from 100 to 1600 cycles per second, a frequency that is higher than any human body frequency that had been previously recorded.

The Intuitive Explanation of Chakras

The chakras, like meridians, receive and carry data on electromagnetic frequencies. Now, while meridians transmit data as a gestalt (a whole pattern), the chakras receive and process only a small range of frequencies that are a part of the whole. The individual chakras, like radio stations, process only selected data. You will come to see that these chakras are highly rapid and efficient data processing systems.

These chakras also act as transformers. Any change in a primary coil's current will induce a voltage in an adjacent coil. Similarly, the energy of a lower chakra radiates to the chakra that is higher up, thereby inducing a surge in voltage that increases the power of the higher chakra. Therefore, chakras act as step-up and step-down transformers.

Now, the process of individual evolution requires that a person heal his or her chakras and their emotional data. It might be seen that people might be repeating the very same self-destructive behavior because they are working with programs that might have not been upgraded since the time they were created. Therefore, it is important to heal both the physical trauma that chakras might experience, as well as the programs that are created to process experiences.

The energetic healing at the hands of an expert can heal the chakras and help one gain valuable insight. The process of energetic healing also serves to stimulate the chakras, thereby increasing the likelihood that the energy flow that results will be powerful enough to open all the major chakras. It is the higher chakras, really, that can give old data new perspectives and insights, and it is these that need to be opened in order to bring that much-needed change.

Therefore, the process of energetic healing can help open the higher chakras, and as the energy moves up and down the chakras, we will gradually leave all that is habitual but no longer serves us. As we heal our chakras, we will find that the old ways in which we interpret and perceive our lives will change, and what was once painful might no longer even be important anymore.

Chapter 15

The Power of Smell – Nursing through Aromatherapy

It is now widely accepted that aromatherapy has a great role to play where it comes to fostering a holistic healing environment for patients. Let's take a look at it in greater detail.

How Aromatherapy Works

The term *aromatherapy* essentially refers to the therapeutic use of essential oils. Essential oils are nothing short of being the volatile organic constituents of plants. It must be noted that these oils are thought to work at *psychological, physiological* and even *cellular*, levels. This implies that they can affect our bodies, minds and even all the delicate links that are in between.

117

The effects of aroma are rapid indeed, and sometimes even thinking about the aroma can be as poignant as the actual smell itself. For instance, try this exercise yourself. Take aside a few moments to think of your favorite scented flower. You can definitely bring an image of it to your mind and almost smell it, right? Doesn't it make you feel peaceful? You will find that the effects of an aroma can be relaxing or even stimulating, depending on the previous experience of the individual (which is also called the 'learned memory'), in addition to the actual chemical makeup of the essential oil that is used.

So, who uses aromatherapy, really? Well, you will come to see that nurses in places like the United Kingdom, Japan and Germany commonly use it. In fact, in France and Germany, medical doctors even use aromatherapy as a part of conventional medicine, where it comes to the process of controlling infection. Believe it or not, it is the fastest-growing therapy among nurses in the United States.

Although in general essential oils are very safe to use, there are some guidelines that need to be followed. There is some evidence of adverse skin reactions that have been caused by sensitivity. In most of these cases, it was on account of extracts that contained topical preservatives, instead of pure essential oils. People with multiple allergies are more likely to be sensitive to aromatherapy, as well.

How is aromatherapy administered?

Essential oils can be used topically or even inhaled. Some essential oils, like lavender and tea tree oil, can be used undiluted topically in the cases of treating stings and bites. Yet others, like clove and thyme, should never be used undiluted on the skin because of their high phenol content, which can cause burns.

Aromatherapy can be very useful to treat insomnia or depression. For instance, a drop of peppermint oil can help clear your mind miraculously, at the end of a stressful day. Lavender can be used most effectively where it comes to the treatment of pain. It is key to take consideration of a few points where it comes to administering aromatherapy effectively. These are things like the client's like and dislike of particular aromas, their perception of the problem and level of stress.

Chapter 16

Communication – The most Therapeutic form of Holistic Nursing

In this chapter, we will touch upon the most vital segment in the field of holistic nursing – *therapeutic communication*.

Therapeutic Communication

Therapeutic communication can be briefly defined as a counseling approach that makes the client's self-discovery the key focus. It is found that through the process of using this approach, a positive, supportive relationship can be developed; one that enables the client to explore the gamut of his or her personal relationships and behavior.

This model of communication entails a style of practice that lays the emphasis on patient empowerment and not on professional control. The client can check the accuracy of the perceptions immediately with the helper, through the use of interpersonal skills. This serves to provide the client with timely and personal feedback, where it comes to personal issues. Following the valuable insights that are gleaned in the process, the client can make the clearest decisions in order to bring about the necessary changes.

You will see that the helper has to use several skills in order to achieve the very best level of therapeutic communication. There are many aspects of the self that are involved in this process, and they include accurate listening, personal awareness, wisdom, knowledge of the change process that is not linear, and intuitive knowing. It has been found that systematic training, as well as the practice of interpersonal skills, helps to increase the self-efficacy of the helper, as far as providing holistic care to the patient is concerned.

Through a more complex cognitive processing, the helper is able to take a point of view that is discrepant from their own, and also able to manage information better. In the process, the personal development of the healer occurs as their very own understanding of their development style, as well as that of others, are highlighted.

There is another key element of helping, and that is keeping the focus on the patient's wholeness, rather than the dysfunctions that he or she clearly exhibits. When there is attention given to the patient as a whole, it allows them the *energetic emphasis* to attain the greatest possible growth. This is contrary to conventional medical practice, where the focus lies on pathology and not on the energetic exchange between healer and client.

Where it comes to ordinary listening, the participants frequently use skills like active listening and questioning. Each participant is fully invested in being heard, as well as sharing his or her unique story. Advice is often solicited as well as given. You will find that in therapeutic communication, the entire focus is on the client. The helper puts his or her feelings and thoughts aside, in order to affirm and assist in clarifying the client's personal expression and meaning. As the relationship develops, the helper guides the client deeper into areas of behavior or patterns, which the client may not be fully aware of themselves.

Therapeutic Communication Skills

It is a given, really, that helpers must master their communication skills in order to provide the best healing care for the patient. Let's take a look at exactly all that this process entails.

The Stages in The building of Therapeutic Communication Skills

Stage One – The Building of the Relationship

In this most pivotal stage, you will find that *empathy* is the first skill that needs to be worked upon, in order for the helper to build the best sense of rapport with the client. It is this very skill that enables the helper to communicate to the client the understanding and acceptance of the client's expressed feelings, as well as the very reason behind those feelings.

You will see that each time a thought is born, a feeling or emotion follows. You will find that in Western society, feelings have been split from content so that only the reasons for the reactions are shared. What empathy strives to do is to reconnect these parts, so that the client can understand the full meaning of what is being shared.

There are several things that the helper must do in order to hear the client accurately. At the very outset, the inner distractions must be avoided so that the helper can listen to what is being said as well as the manner in which it is being said. The dominant feeling of the client is then identified, and the reasons for that feeling are ascertained. The helper will then strive to respond with fresh words that reflect the same meaning as those offered by the client in a concise and incisive manner.

The second core skill that needs to be used in this stage of therapeutic communication is *respect*. Of course, we all know by now that each client is a unique individual who is a precious whole being. The helper has to see various ailments, the client might be suffering from, as a whole in order to actualize their highest potential. One of the greatest things that the helper can give their client is self-respect. The clients usually know the things that are important –things that are required for their healing. What the helpers should do is to encourage the virtue of self-determination in them.

The process of acknowledging one's self-resources is a great way to build self-respect. You will find that patients who are wrapped up in their problems lose sight of the valuable resources that are needed in order to deal with the situation. Here you will find that gentle reminders of skills that are used to cope with problems current or past, can help greatly where it comes to reinforcing the client's coping skills.

The next virtue that is important where it comes to this stage is that of *genuineness.* This goes a long way in leading the helper to present himself or herself as a human being, and not merely a role. Using this virtue, the helper might share some feelings with the client. For instance, if the client is stuck on discussing a particular issue, the helper might tell him or her that they have been there before and what is of paramount importance is what they are feeling in the given moment.

The next virtue is that of concreteness. It includes important things like *purposeful questioning* and *summarization.* You will find that purposeful questioning is used when the client's answers are vague. Very often you will find that a client will disguise an important issue, by using a word to signify a larger issue. Here you will find that using the words *how, what, when* and *describe,* encourages the clients to further detail what it is they are experiencing. Here it must be noted that the word why should not be used because it requires the client to have a complete understanding of what has happened.

Stage Two: Deeper Exploration

In this stage, there are five skills that are used: *additive empathy, self-disclosure, feedback, confrontation*, and *immediacy*. In this stage, you will find that the client's deeper patterns are revealed, and they come to acknowledge how these patterns are maintained. Here you will find that the helper provides a wider view than the client can see within the very own perspective of their life.

Let us explore all the skills of this stage, one by one.

Additive empathy. Using this skill, the helper listens for and describes the underlying feelings and behavioral themes. Usually, you will find that the clients are themselves not aware of their underlying feelings. The process of bringing these skills to the surface gives the chance to the client to see exactly how they operate, and whether or not to continue them. So, how does this process work? There are three things that need to be explored where it comes to this skill.

> Focusing on the surface and deeper feelings, as well as the underlying fears.

> Identifying the themes and the patterns of response that the client normally uses.

> Identifying the client's personalization of the pattern

Self-disclosure. Here the helper uses his or her own life experience to help in the process.

It becomes vital to match the feeling area and to deepen the sharing of underlying fears, even though the life situation of the healer might be intrinsically different from that of the client. This skill helps expertly, where it comes to taking the clients back to their very own process of self-discovery.

Feedback. This is a skill that is fairly familiar, one that provides a great deal of information to the client. To make sure this skill is developed to the very best of one's abilities, one must ensure that they bear in mind that the primordial motivation for sharing information is to *assist* the other person.

They need to define specific behaviors that need to be changed and make no assumptions or interpretations of the behavior of the client. It's also about conveying the impact of the behavior on others, and giving feedback directly to the client when the behavior occurs. Lastly, it's about ensuring that the client is in a receptive mode to hear the feedback in the very first instance.

Confrontation. This skill invites the clients to examine discrepancies in their behavior – in what is said, felt, thought and finally, done. You will find that some of these behaviors might be in the consciousness of these clients, while some might not. The client might initially deny the truth of the information. It is then the role of the healer to gently repeat this information in fresh words after the client has been acknowledged for the reaction through the use of primary empathy.

Immediacy. This skill deals with exploring the relationship at the current moment in time. The times when immediacy is important are when the client's psychological needs and intentions try to influence the helper to take on a certain role that will satisfy those very needs. It is important to note here that the client might not be aware of this influencing behavior, so bringing it into awareness can be very helpful for self-discovery and healing.

Stage 3: Implementation

In this final stage of therapeutic communication, the idea is to implement the things for which the groundwork has already been laid thus far. This is the problem-solving stage of the model and one of the most important stages where it comes to bringing about that actual change in the client's life.

The very first step here is to clarify the exact goal. The helper must help the client set a goal that is *appropriate*. It can be helpful here to ask questions pertaining to what the client wants right now, and what they want next year. Also, can the client support this goal one hundred percent and what might they do to sabotage this goal?

No matter what the goals laid in the end are, they need to be specific enough for the client to recognize the accomplishment of each one. In fact, one of the guidelines in setting these goals would be to ask if these goals would be visible, concrete and specific enough to be observed by others. Then, once a clear goal is set, the various options for the client should be considered.

Often you will come to see that the client sees only one or two goals, which he or she in all probability might have already tried. Here is where the process of brainstorming is important so that the helper and client can come up with several possible ways in meeting those goals.

Finally, when the list is completed, the client should choose three alternatives that are most *appealing* as well as *workable*, of course. Then, the client should evaluate all alternatives using a cost-gain analysis, in order to see which one to use first. Once an alternative has been zoned in on as being the one of primary choice, steps can be taken to reach the goal.

Chapter 17

The Holistic Nursing and Caring Process

Let us take a deeper look at the holistic caring process, now, and see all that it enunciates in its deepest essence.

The Holistic Caring Process

The *Holistic Caring Process* is nothing short of being an adaptation and expansion of the nursing process that incorporates the holistic nursing philosophy. On closer observation, you will come to see that it is a systematic, dynamic and living framework that is used for discovering, describing and documenting the health patterns that are unique to a person.

You will come to see that these patterns, that are identified within the nurse-person relationship, lay the foundation for the mutual goals and the responses to actions initiated in the nurse-person caring process.

As we have already touched upon several times over the course of this book, the contemporary definition of nursing, which comes from the *American Nurses' Association*, incorporates the concept of caring for the whole person. There are four essential features of practice, where this definition Of nursing is concerned. They are the following.

> The attention to the full range of human experiences and the responses to health and illness without any sort of restriction to a problem-focused orientation.

> The integration of objective data with the knowledge that is gained from the understanding of the person's or the group's subjective experience.

> The application of scientific knowledge to the processes of diagnosis and treatment.

> Finally, the provision of a caring relationship; one that strives to facilitate health and healing.

You will find that while it is focused on the health and wellbeing within a person, the holistic caring process is circular in nature and includes the following six steps: *assessment, patterns / challenges / needs, outcomes, therapeutic care plan, implementation, and evaluation.*

The original concept of the holistic caring process can be traced way back to the late 1950s and the early 1960s when nursing in the United States of America sought to identify itself as a distinct and autonomous profession within healthcare. It was none other than *Kreuter*, who first identified the formalization of the nursing process as an orderly approach to the conduct of independent nursing activities in the year 1957.

I noted that there were two definitions for the nursing caring process. The first went on to define it as a step-by-step linear process for solving problems. The second one, one that is more compatible with the holistic caring process as we know it today, sought to define it as a means of reflecting on the entire process of client-nurse interaction.

In due course of time, the circular view of the nursing process faded when the very first nursing definition of the nursing process as a problem-solving model that was based on the scientific method became the definition that was generally accepted. In fact, this model was unquestionably the model that laid the foundation for nursing practice and education until the early 1980s, when nursing scholars began to focus on philosophy and theory in nursing.

Pattern recognition

The very origins of the nursing process reside in the concept of *pattern recognition*, which is an innate tendency found amongst many humans. You will come to see that pattern recognition can be seen even in young infants, who come to recognize and react to patterns in their caregivers, that are both familiar as well as unfamiliar. These patterns can be facial, vocal or even kinesthetic in nature.

The very first thing that nurses observe when they come in contact with a patient for the very first time, is the state of the patient's health. They observe the patient's color (whether it is pale or cyanotic), their affect and eye contact, as well as their respiration rate and volume of speech, apart from their bodily scars and wounds, amongst other things. It is within the span of 60 seconds itself that they come to notice if something is different from the expected and if any nursing action is necessary or not. This is the process of *pattern appraisal and pattern recognition*.

You will come to see that using all their vast resources of nursing knowledge, nurses apply the patterns that they observe to known patterns, make decisions about those very patterns and then act upon those decisions. After doing so, they reappraise and react based upon the response of the person.

Also, this nursing process is culturally shaped and is inseparable from the culture in which it is practiced. Since in concept the nursing process cannot be separated from the cultural context in which it is practiced, the holistic nurse must embrace this concept when implementing theory-based practice. The holistic nurses that work within the contemporary health care culture must balance formal knowledge and expertise that are gained from nursing education and practice, along with philosophies of health that might not yet be embraced fully by mainstream culture.

You will come to see, on closer observation, that the holistic caring practice is established upon *reflective practice*. The insights that have been derived from the four patterns of knowing, that have been established by

132

Carper, guide the process of the nurse within the nurse-person interaction. The empirical or scientific knowledge is based on the *objective information* that is measurable by the senses and by the process of scientific instrumentation.

Aesthetic knowledge, on the other hand, draws on a sense of form and structure, and of beauty and creativity, in order to discern patterns and change.

Personal knowledge strives to incorporate the nurses' self-awareness and knowledge, as well as the intuitive perceptions of meanings that are based on personal experiences. This is in fact demonstrated effectively through the therapeutic use of self.

Thus, the nurses who adhere to the holistic caring process tenets, focus on the care of the whole unique person, while at the very same time championing the patient's rights to the very best of their abilities. Based on a thorough holistic assessment as well as an identification of the patient's health patterns, the decisions about the care flow through the collaboration with the person, other health care providers, and significant others.

Therefore, it is clear that the person themselves goes on to assume an important role in the healthcare planning as well as decision making, through the process of seeking professional expertise from the nurse via the various nurse-person interactions. You will find that, facilitated by the nurse in the healing relationship, the person expresses health concerns and strengths that the nurse identifies and documents in the health care record.

Thus, the person is encouraged to participate as actively as possible, taking responsibility for his or her health choices as well as decisions for self-care.

One of the most important things for nurses to remember is this: that the process of holistic caring is merely a tool; a framework for ordering, documenting and discussing the nurse-person interactions. Excessive reliance on structure and objectivity might, in turn, reduce the person to nothing short of being an object themselves.

Assessment

This is another integral part of the holistic caring process. As we have touched upon earlier, this is the information gathering phase in which the nurse and the person identify health patterns as well as prioritize the person's healthcare concerns. This is a continuous process and it provides the ongoing data for changes that occur over the course of time. You will come to see that each nurse-person encounter provides vital new information that helps to explain the interrelationships as well as validates the previously collected data and conclusions.

You will find that a key to a holistic assessment is to appraise the overall pattern of the responses. The nurse uncovers the information about the person's patterns, through the processes of interaction, observation, and measurement. You will find that each pattern identification taps into the hologram of the person. The interpersonal interaction between the person and the nurse, reveals the perceptions, feelings, and thoughts about the health patterns as identified by the person.

It has come to be seen that nursing observation relies on information that is perceived by the five senses, as well as intuition, while the process of measurement provides quantifiable information that can be revealed by scientific instruments. You will find that the client is the primary source and the interpreter of the meaning of the information that is obtained from the assessment sources.

Furthermore, there is supplemental information that is provided by members of the family, significant others, other health care professionals as well as measurable data. You will see that within the cultural context of negotiation, this vital phase of assessment might be seen as an exchange of expert knowledge wherein both the nurse and the person bring expertise to the exchange.

It is within the assessment of the person's *bio-pyscho-social-spiritual patterns* that the nurse looks for the overall pattern of interrelationships. He or she uses the appropriate scientific and intuitive approaches, assesses the state of the energy field, and identifies the stages of change as well as the readiness to change. The nurse also collects pivotal client data from the previous nursing records, if any, as well as other members of the healthcare team, if appropriate. All of the pertinent data are documented in the person's record.

Thus, the holistic nurses views the person as a whole and listens for the meaning of the current health situation, to the person within the environment. While acknowledging their own patterns and their potential influence on the healing relationship, the nurse reflects on the patient's patterns that have been gleaned from the assessment. In tandem, the person validates the patterns that have been recognized from the assessment.

You will find that the processes of assessment and documentation are continuous, where it comes to the nurse-person relationship. This is because changes in one pattern always lead to some change in the other dimension. If there is a lack of awareness about one's own beliefs and patterns, it might significantly influence the nurse-client relationship. For instance, communication barriers are relative to class, culture, age, gender, etcetera. Thereby, a holistic assessment might be impaired in the process.

Intuitive Thinking

The process of intuitive thinking is also integral to the holistic caring process. This is important because the process of holistically assessing the status of a person involves the evaluation of data not only from a rational, analytic mode, but also from an intuitive, nonverbal mode.

Unfortunately, intuitive perceptions have been seen as striving to oppose the empirical knowledge base of practice. The good news, however, is the fact that things are changing. People are coming to see that it is not only *quantifiable data* that is important anymore. The good part is that intuitive thinking does not clash with the process of analytic reasoning. Simply put, it is another *dimension of knowing*. There are multiple ways of knowing and assessing the status of clients, and this intuitive process is most integral to the nursing process.

There is a qualitative yet indefinable process that scientists use to organize fragments of findings into meaningful wholes. This very indefinable process is known as intuition –a process through which people know more than they can explain.

The process of intuitive perception allows a person to know something immediately without the conscious use of reason. Clinical intuition has been defined as *'a process by which we know something about a client which cannot be verbalized or is verbalized poorly or for which the source of knowledge cannot be determined.'* In essence, really, it is nothing short of being a gut feeling that something is wrong or that we should do something, even if there is no evidence to support that feeling.

You will come to see that the most experienced and technically skilled nurses have been found to be highly intuitive thinkers. It is within the most caring relationship between the nurse and the person that intuitive events emerge. This is largely on account of the fact that the nurse is open and receptive to the subtle cues of the person, such as color, activity, and posture.

Acknowledging and dismissing fear

Let us discuss what exactly fear is in the very first place, and where it comes from. You will find that it is this very fear that can surface when we contemplate lifestyle changes. Let's take a simple example. A person who wishes to stop smoking is scared of giving up his or her longheld habit, simply because they fear that they might have severe withdrawal symptoms, gain weight and perhaps even offend people by asking them not to smoke.

Thus, you will come to see that this fear will surface only in relation to something else. So, how can we gain freedom from this very sense of fear? In fact, this is a pivotal part of the healing process – the process of learning more about fear in relation to all things.

The thing is, there are times when fear can actually attach itself to the spirit and lodge itself somewhere in the body. There are times when it can make us feel alone beyond comprehension, but the good news is that it can become a path that will actually lead us deeper into the present moment. Even though the fact remains that fear can create more fear, its very occurrence can be a moment to learn about an intrinsic part of life's journey.

The good thing about fear is the fact that it can make us pay our attention to the areas in which we have some form of resistance. It is through the process of releasing this very fear that we can return to our core of unconditional love so that we can release all the 'shoulds' that have been clouding our vision for way too long.

The very basic fears of rejection, the unknown and failure, are closely related and might overlap. You will come to see that any kind of fear is really related to our level of self-esteem. Our fears tend to increase when our levels of self-esteem are low. The kind of negative self-talk that we indulge in whilst in the throes of fear only serves to dampen our levels of self-confidence and takes us even further away from the resolution of fear.

In an attempt to identify our stressors and the role that they play where it comes to evoking our fears, we need to ask ourselves the following questions.

How do I usually react to my fears? Am I the kind of person that hopes that the very circumstances that are surrounding the fear will go away?

Is there anyone of the basic human fears that tends to dominate my list of stressors? If so, what is the cause behind it?

What are the strategies that I can use to deal with some of my major fears?

You will come to see that through the process of asking these most pivotal questions, you come to embrace your fears in the process and it is through this very acknowledgment, that one can begin the process of quelling their fears so that they can take their healing process to the next level.

Conclusion

We have seen over the course of this book, all that holistic nursing entails. We have come to see that the process of holistic healing is really a synergistic approach, where it comes to harnessing the well being of the trinity of mind, body, and spirit.

Holistic nursing goes beyond mere nursing. In fact, the shift to the wellness model has prompted the profession to take a new look at research priorities, methodologies, and findings. We have seen how holistic nurses are committed to the process of empowering the client. The use of the holistic approach provides the client with a powerful way to be instrumental in their self-healing.

The fact remains, there is a tremendous emphasis on 'doing' in the Western World, where we are judged by our capacity to *do things* rather than to *just be*. The thing is, though, that illness takes away a patient's capacity to do things and forces him or her to address their being on a much larger scale. However frightening this might be, it allows the holistic nurse to present to the patient the view of a multidimensional world that has hitherto remained hidden as far as the patient is concerned.

We have come to see that holistic nursing is a process that is far more intuitive than one might have thought. Rather than depending on facts and figures, it relies heavily on the ability to sense things that cannot be evaluated in the conventional sense. We have also seen that the process of holistic nursing, while extremely beneficial to the patient, is also of great benefit to the person providing that holistic care. It is a symbiotic relationship between the nurse and the patient, one that helps both of them grown in the process.

The process of holistic nursing is here to stay, and will only get better over the time to come. People will come to see that it is the human spirit that is really most powerful, and that is what needs to be focused on in addition to treating the body and mind. This is the very reason that hospitals need to invest in people as their bottom line, with a view to optimizing the hospital experience for the patient.

We need to realize that a healing environment begins by acknowledging that the current hospital environment emphasizes *curing* and not *healing*. A real effort is required where it comes to determining the individual needs of the hospital, the patient population as well as the staff. It is through the use of centering and intentionality that the holistic nurse can become a healing environment and participate in the creation of a healing healthcare system that integrates both masculine and feminine attributes.

In the end, it is safe to say that holistic nursing is as much *Art as it is Science*. The intent of artistic nursing is healing, and that is, in essence, a spiritual process.

One last thing!

I want to give you a **one-in-two-hundred chance** to win a **$200.00 Amazon Gift card** as a thank-you for reading this book.

All I ask is that you give me some feedback, so I can improve this or my next book :)

Your opinion is *super valuable* to me. It will only take a minute of your time to let me know what you like and what you didn't like about this book. The hardest part is deciding how to spend the two hundred dollars! Just follow this link.

http://reviewers.win/holisticnursing

Made in United States
Orlando, FL
12 October 2023